CREATING WHOLENESS

A Self-Healing Workbook
Using Dynamic Relaxation,
Images, and Thoughts

CREATING WHOLENESS

A Self-Healing Workbook
Using Dynamic Relaxation,
Images, and Thoughts

31030 1

Erik Peper

San Francisco State University
San Francisco, California

and

Catherine F. Holt

Biofeedback and Family Therapy Institute
Berkeley, California

Plenum Press • New York and London

Library of Congress Cataloging-in-Publication Data

Peper, Erik.
    Creating wholeness : a self-healing workbook using relaxation,
  images, and thoughts / Erik Peper and Catherine F. Holt.
        p.   cm.
    Includes bibliographical references and index.
    ISBN 0-306-44172-1
    1. Holistic medicine. 2. Self-care, Health.   I. Holt, Catherine
  F. II. Title.
    [DNLM: 1. Holistic Health. 2. Imagination. 3. Relaxation.
  4. Self Care. 5. Thinking.   WB 545 P421c]
  R733.P46 1993
  613--dc20
  DNLM/DLC
  for Library of Congress   92-48857
                                                                 CIP

10 9 8 7 6 5

This book is not a substitute for medical advice. For such advice, consult
a health care professional.

ISBN 0-306-44172-1

© 1993 Plenum Press, New York
A Division of Plenum Publishing Corporation
233 Spring Street, New York, N.Y. 10013

Printed in the United States of America

Preface

This workbook grew out of the practices assigned for self-growth and development for (1) Holistic Health: Western Perspectives, a course at San Francisco State University; (2) clients and participants at the Biofeedback and Family Therapy Institute in Berkeley; and (3) participants in peak performance training programs. The goals of this workbook are to offer experiences to facilitate life-long learning of skills to enhance health and growth.

We hope the reader will experience increased autonomy and gain self-mastery skills through exercises that foster awareness and control. The cascading program is based upon uncovering, allowing, and encouraging the intrinsic drive toward integration, wholeness, and health. Each year many of our students report that practicing these skills has affected them deeply. The program offered them pragmatic skills to master stress, set goals, and experience a deep change in their worldview and health. A number of them have said that this was the most useful course they had taken at San Francisco State University.

The materials presented here are part of a course offered by the Institute for Holistic Healing Studies. It is also a requirement for a Holistic Health Minor and fulfills a part of the general education requirement for integrated and interdisciplinary learning. The development of this program at San Francisco State University is due to the foresight and courage of George Araki, Ph.D.

Acknowledgments

This workbook would not have been possible without the honest and sometimes even painful feedback of the students. We feel privileged to have had the opportunity to read their responses and papers that developed from these practices. We want to thank many students for participating in our exploration. They have been outstanding teachers by sharing the wisdom they acquired through their process of self-healing. Their feedback was of great assistance in the shaping of this workbook. We specifically thank the following people for allowing us to quote from their papers: Cie-jae Allen, Collet Campbell, Lisa Green, Wendy Hussey, Janice Mettler, Gayathri Perera, and Susan Wilson.

We thank Vicci Tibbetts for her many constructive recommendations and Lesli Fullerton for her careful reading of the early versions of the manuscript and helpful suggestions. We also thank Louisa Howe, Charles Lynch, Jackie Benson, Alex Pierce, Denis DiBartolomeo, and Carol Aronoff for their comments. We also thank Eliot Werner and Herman Makler of Plenum Press for helping to make the book a reality.

We appreciate the support and patience of close family members who had to put up with us as we increased their stress while we worked on the book. We thank Karen for her continued support and love while we labored.

The selected quotes on pages 3, 31, 33, 47, 114, 118, 141, 161, and 183 are reprinted from *Words to Live By: Inspiration for Every Day,* by Eknath Easwaran, with permission of Nilgiri Press.

Contents

4. Self-Healing Through Imagery and Behavior Change   159

Appendix: Audiotapes and Temperature Monitoring Devices   215

Notes   217

References   219

Suggested Readings on Holistic Health   221

Index   225

Chapter 1
Introduction

There is a point of consciousness within everyone which has the seed of wholeness. By wholeness I mean the potential to realize integration within oneself, and to actively direct the forces of one's life . . .

Dora Van Gelder Kunz

SYSTEMS PERSPECTIVE OF HEALTH

The hipbone's connected to the thighbone, the thighbone's connected to the legbone . . .
                                                                    TRADITIONAL SONG

A human being is part of the whole, called by us "universe," a part limited in time and space. He experiences himself, has thoughts and feelings, as something separate from the rest—a kind of optical delusion of consciousness. This delusion is a kind of prison for us, restricting us to our personal desires and to affection for a few persons nearest to us. Our task must be to free ourselves from this prison by widening our circles of compassion to embrace all living creatures and the whole of nature in its beauty.
                                                                    ALBERT EINSTEIN

A basic premise of holistic health is a systems perspective in which every part in a system affects and is affected by every other part. We are embedded in and part of the whole. In the words of John Donne, "No man is an island, entire of itself; every man is a piece of the continent, a part of the main." This means that how we use ourselves (live our lives) affects our structure and our structure affects how we use ourselves.

Our health is the integration of multiple components that influence and augment each other. The factors that affect our health include, among others, genetics[1], family and socioeconomic background, diet, exercise, social support, risk-taking behaviors, attitude, and spiritual practices. All these factors affect our present and future health. It is important to remember that these components are not separate. A holistic approach to health recognizes the interconnectedness of body, mind, spirit, and environment. This systems view perceives the individual as a powerful creator of his or her own health, able to make conscious choices about nutrition, exercise, social and career paths, thoughts and images. In regaining control over your own health, some important tools will be the following: relaxation, diaphragmatic breathing, cognitive stress reduction, and imagery for healing and behavior change. A major theme linking all these components is the importance of mindfulness; that is, the integration of your awareness and skills into everyday life situations.

Regardless of how healthy or ill we are, we can be an active partner in our own growth. Arthur Frank (1991), who had a heart attack at age 39 and cancer the following year, stated in his book *At the Will of the Body*, "Illness takes away parts of your life, but in doing so it gives you the opportunity to choose the life you will lead, as opposed to living out the one you have simply accumulated over the years." (p. 1)

The focus of this workbook is to help you choose the kind of life you will lead. We offer some strategies that will help you begin to become an active participant in your growth/health process. It will cover only a few of the many factors that we believe affect our health. We hope to offer support to "nature's self-directed growth process." This sense of support for growth is radically different from the more traditional health care—or, actually, illness care—system.

At times, people have made a reductionistic comparison between our soma (body/mind structure and process) and a car. If something is wrong with a car, you just fix it by repairing the carburetor or getting a valve job. If you have heart disease you get a plastic heart valve or a venous graft for coronary artery bypass surgery. Continuing this analogy, your body could be like an underpowered car, with a poor transmission and worn tires. Yet you can nurture the car for a long time by driving carefully and avoiding jack rabbit starts and stops, hills, and potholes; that is, you would maximize the potential in the situation.

The preceding analogy is faulty because the human being is NOT a mechanical, nonregenerative machine. The human being is a generative process. Depending on how you use yourself, you may regenerate and grow. Imagine a regenerating and evolving car: If you took good care of your car, the tires would regenerate and develop more tread. This growth potential is inherent in our soma. Within our soma there is an intrinsic drive toward integration and wholeness. We are an energy flow that can only go forward. We cannot go back to being the same as we were yesterday any more than a flowing river can go back to containing yesterday's water. Not to change is unhealthy and abnormal, since the nature of our being is continuous change, flux, and growth.

This workbook is designed for use either on your own, with a guide or therapist, or as part of a class. You could also create an informal "relaxation and self-healing group." This workbook focuses on encouraging and allowing this intrinsic drive toward health. Health and its concurrent quality of life are multidimensional.

Multiple Factors Create Health

Health is far more than the absence of illness or symptoms. It goes beyond the condition of the physical body and includes emotional, mental, and spiritual factors. We can no longer separate the emotional state from the physical state, since every thought or feeling leaves its traces on the body. As Elmer and Alyce Green (1977), two well-known pioneers in the field of biofeedback, wrote, "Every change in the physiological state is accompanied by an appropriate change in the mental–emotional state, conscious or unconscious, and every change in the mental–emotional state, conscious or unconscious, is accompanied by an appropriate change in the physiological state."

Often, factors in our lifestyles become interwoven. If you feel depressed, you may think, "What's the point?" when it comes to exercise. If you feel overburdened with work, you may decide there's just no time for fun or relaxation. If you are depriving yourself of sleep, caffeine and sugar may seem necessary to get you through the day. If you have chronic pain, you may isolate yourself from people. Such circumstances can make change seem difficult, or even impossible—especially if you see many areas out of balance. The good news about these connections, however, is this: No matter where you start, a positive change in one area often sets off a number of other beneficial changes that flow almost effortlessly. For example, exercise can regulate appetite, improve self-esteem, give you more energy, and even alleviate pain; it may enhance your social support network, too, as you meet others in a yoga class, in a swimming pool, or at a gym.

Since it doesn't really matter where you start, you can choose the step that is the easiest, smallest, and most enjoyable for you. As you achieve success with your modest goal, your motivation level is sure to build. One woman realized that she had gotten into the habit of overeating to comfort herself for the loss of a dance class. For her weight-loss program, finding a new dance class turned out to be more important than counting calories. As she began dancing, she stopped feeling deprived and automatically ate less. A woman with daily headaches and work overload had stopped calling friends and socializing. She chose to start smiling at strangers and seeing her friends more often, and the headaches disappeared. The self-healing process has a life of its own.

Although it may not be immediately obvious, for many people a connection with nature can be very healing for the body, mind, and spirit. Even doing something positive for the planet, like recycling, seems to have a beneficial effect. Breathing the pure air in the mountains makes us less inclined to eat junk food.

> I pledge allegiance to the Earth:
> I will honor this body given me by birth.
> The body is my connection with the Mother;
> If I pollute one, then I pollute the other.
> The unity of body and mind
> Brings peace and wisdom to humankind.
> CATHY HOLT

This workbook will not give you specific information on what constitutes the best diet, exercise program, and so on. We believe there is plenty of literature about those fitness areas (see Recommended Readings). Rather, we hope to provide a useful guide to help you overcome your obstacles and begin on your self-designed path to greater well-being.

As a starting point, it is good to be aware of where you are with respect to the larger picture of health-supporting behaviors and environment. Look over the following twelve health areas to get a sense of where your assets and liabilities are. How might you bring more balance into your life? Where might you like to start?

12 Factors Promoting Health

1. Healthful diet
   - Chiefly whole foods, such as fruits, vegetables, whole grains
   - Three meals a day
   - At least one hot balanced meal daily
   - Breakfast every day
   - Low fat
   - Low salt
   - Low sugar
   - Low meat consumption (eat low on food chain)
   - Few processed foods or food additives

2. No smoking

3. Little or no caffeine
   - Fewer than three cups of caffeinated coffee or black tea or cola drinks per day

4. Little or no alcohol
   - Fewer than four alcoholic drinks per week

5. Appropriate weight
   - Neither obese nor anorexic
   - Comfortable about your weight

6. Regular exercise
   - Some form of aerobic exercise at least three times a week
   - Stretching
   - Having plenty of energy

7. Regular relaxation
   - Quiet time/time alone daily
   - Time for play or fun at least once a week
   - Time in nature

8. Adequate sleep
   - 7–8 hours of sleep per night
   - Feeling refreshed from sleep

9. Safety habits
   - Car seat belt/air bags
   - Motorcycle helmet
   - Nonhazardous working environment
   - Safe, nontoxic living environment

10. Resolution of anger/resentment/fear daily
    - No "unfinished business"
    - Regular conversations about domestic issues with those you live with
    - Ability to express feelings
    - Ability to say no without guilt

11. Positive attitude
    - Liking, nurturing, and doing nice things for yourself
    - Finding your work or studies rewarding and challenging
    - Being comfortable with your income
    - Perceiving problems as opportunities for growth
    - Seeing the humor in everything
    - Drawing strength from spiritual beliefs

12. Social support system
    - Network of friends/acquaintances/relatives
    - Giving and receiving hugs and affection regularly (at least four hugs a day!)
    - Having at least one friend to confide in
    - Ability to ask for help when needed
    - Being a good listener
    - Feeling content with your level of intimacy and sexual activity

**12 Steps to Health:
A Summary**

1. Healthful diet
2. No smoking
3. Little or no caffeine
4. Little or no alcohol
5. Appropriate weight
6. Regular exercise
7. Regular relaxation
8. Adequate sleep
9. Safety habits
10. Resolution of anger/resentment/fear daily
11. Positive attitude
12. Social support system

HOW TO GET THE MOST OUT OF THIS WORKBOOK

> QUESTION: *"How many psychologists does it take to change a light bulb?"*
> ANSWER: *"One, but only if it really wants to change."*

This workbook demands active participation. The more you put into it—the more you practice—the more you will gain. Learning awareness, relaxation, stress management, acceptance and control over thoughts and emotions takes time. It is in the practice and actual experience that change occurs. Although many of our students have reported benefits when they practice only a few times, most report that the process of awareness, change and growth is similar to developing or learning any new skill.

Many of you know that it took weeks to master driving a car. Remember when you first learned? It took all your concentration to drive down the street. It seemed almost overwhelming to attend simultaneously to other cars, pedestrians, traffic signs, steering the car, pressing the gas pedal or brake and also pushing the clutch down and shifting gears. Most of you now drive while talking to someone, playing with the radio, dialing a number on the car telephone, or observing the scenery. In fact, sometimes you now get to your destination without remembering ever driving there. How did you shift from this intense concentration and attention to allowing the driving to be automatic? A major component is PRACTICE. To benefit from this workbook the role is similar: *Through practice you reap the benefits.*

We recommend that you first glance through the exercises and then sequentially practice them. Generally, the exercises each week build upon those of previous weeks, although to some extent they can be done out of order. Practice each exercise daily for at least one week. It usually takes a few days to get used to the practices; after a while they become more automatic. You may find that it takes longer to master some exercises than others. This is normal. Give yourself more time before going on. In addition, you may integrate some components of the practices into your daily routine so that they slowly become part of you.

Even though we all know that we benefit by making changes, we may find that we hesitate to start, pause in the middle, or even stop. There is nothing wrong with that; it is a common experience. Resistance to change is natural. Changing requires energy. We may fear the unknown: "What if this relaxation stuff opens up a Pandora's box of those things I don't want to remember or feel?" We may also fear failure: "What if I set out to heal myself and I don't succeed? Then I'll blame myself and feel worse!" We may even think, "I'm barely keeping it together now, and If I change anything, I might fall apart!" or "My spouse [significant other] won't love me if I change."

Resistance to change usually coexists with a will or desire to change. It is as if there are two personalities battling it out inside us: one that fears and resists change and one that welcomes and seeks it. In order to move forward, it is important to acknowledge and accept the part that is fearful, while not giving in to it. Where did that part come from?

Most of us went through some difficult and frightening times as small children and developed various strategies that allowed us to survive. These strategies may no longer be useful in the present. Often, however, we continue to apply the same strategies even though the situation and the rules have changed as we have matured and grown. As an analogy, consider the training of a baby elephant in a circus. An average rope secured to a small stake in the ground is enough to prevent the little fellow from wandering off; he tests it a few times and learns he is unable to pull it up. Years later, the same flimsy rope and stake are enough to hold the enormous adult elephant, who doesn't bother to test it because he has already learned, as a baby, that it is stronger than he is. Children, too, may learn lasting but self-limiting lessons.

For example, all children have heard their parents criticize or scold their behavior: "You shouldn't do that!" They then learn to criticize themselves and stop the behavior, which earns them love and approval from their parents. However, if they grow up being extremely critical of themselves, they may suffer from anxiety, low self-esteem, and poor self-confidence.

You may decide to explore or change your patterns. However, please welcome and respect them; they are part of you. Many seemingly self-destructive patterns were constructive for you at one time. For example, a lot of people tell themselves that they should exercise, yet they somehow do not find the time to do it. How could this be, since everyone knows exercise is good for us? Actually, for many people exercise is *not* just associated with feeling fit, hard work, and muscle pain. It is also associated with failure. Failure is the covert message often received when we participate in sports. Most competitive sports are designed to have one winner; everyone else fails. Who remembers the silver or bronze medalist in the Olympics? Even in team sports the glory belongs to the team that won—not to the many players who were defeated and lost. It is not only the culture but also our parents who may fail to reward (or may covertly punish) the nonwinner. Because we were sometimes (or may still be) the projections of our parents' dreams, they were disappointed if we didn't win. Hence, it is not surprising that many people with the best of intentions to exercise drop out. Who really wants to reexperience the failure and disappointment so embedded in the past experience of participating in a sport?

Similarly, some people may have difficulty stopping smoking. Again, we believe that stopping is most likely more painful than continuing. How can that be? Isn't smoking bad for you? The answer is probably yes; however, it may fulfill a need even though the person may be unaware of it. For example, lighting a cigarette or taking a puff may give some people a momentary pause before they have to react socially; it gives them time to collect themselves. For others, it may have involved the important process of developing autonomy, which each person needs to develop a sense of self. Smoking can be a statement of autonomy, providing an experience of being in charge and in control: "I am independent of my parents, and there is nothing they can do about it." Hence, if smoking is discontinued, what happens to the sense of self?

As you begin the process of self-exploration and change, be accepting of yourself. Trust that your patterns were meaningful for you and allowed you to survive at some point in the past. You may want to continue and change yet at times want to give up and avoid changing for a while. Accept, comfort, and reassure the part of you that is fearful, just as an adult would comfort a frightened child.

General Guidelines

1. Leisurely scan the workbook to get a flavor of the themes. Observe how the practices change and develop over time. Before embarking on the practices, read the introductory chapter in its entirety. Give special attention to the sections entitled "Some Precautions" and "Important Variables to Optimize Training."

2. Read the instructions for each practice in detail. There is a written script that guides you through each relaxation or imagery practice. We encourage you to adapt the words or sequences in the script to yourself. To lead yourself through each script, it will be helpful for you to make your own audiotape.[2] Detailed instructions are given in the section "Making Your Own Tapes." Each of you is different and unique and will respond in your individual way. As Collet Campbell, a junior at San Francisco State University, wrote: "It is a highly individualized process. It requires complete objectivity in observing *when* and *how* we respond. It requires experimentation and allowances for problems/mistakes in order to discover what works in facilitating positive change."

3. Plan to set aside 20–30 minutes a day to do each practice, plus additional time to make tapes.

4. Record your experiences after you practice each day, and at the end of the week review, integrate, and summarize your experiences. We are often unaware of gradual changes. It is only when our experiences are recorded and reviewed later that we can become aware of the patterns or problems and the changes and growth that we have achieved or allowed. These written records can provide evidence that desired changes are indeed occurring even though, subjectively, we may feel that we have not progressed.

5. At the end of each major chapter of the workbook, look back over the previous weeks' experiences. Summarize your experience to facilitate integration and appreciation of your growth.

6. Be sure to practice the short exercises during the day at home and at work. Integrate those short practices into your life pattern. Just thinking about the practice during the day can be the first step. It may offer a momentary distance from habitual patterns. Just being aware is a significant beginning.

7. If possible, do the exercises together with others in a small group each week. Have family members, friends, or colleagues at work do them with you. Group support is very helpful. In addition, sharing in other people's experiences will augment your own experience and growth. Have a different group member lead and guide the members through the practice each week. If others in your life are not participating or even frown upon your practice, let that be their experience. Don't force them to participate with you, and don't allow their disapproval to defeat you. Remember, each of us has the right to his or her own judgments.

8. If you are part of a group or class, share your findings and discuss your successes and challenges. Have a group member lead you through the next prac-

tice. At the end of the guided session, share your experiences so that you can adapt or change the practice to benefit you most. Remember, when you share in a group, respect each person's experience. In the beginning many people are overly concerned about "doing it right." Do not judge yourself or others. There may be similarities or differences in people's experiences. Give each other support for practicing.

9. If you have difficulty, stop for a few days, then start again with the same or a previous exercise. Sometimes you may want to skip a specific practice and come back to it later. Respect your own process. If something does not seem to work for you, attempt it once more and then *do something different*. If you resist doing the practices, you may want to be like a detective. You might choose to do a detailed analysis of the benefits of NOT doing the practice. Ask yourself, "What are the consequences and rewards for not allowing something new to occur?" Sometimes all it takes is to prioritize our tasks and set up rewards (positive reinforcers) for following through.

10. Do not expect instant success, and do not beat yourself up if you do not attain what you were seeking. Be patient and enjoy the self-discovery. The skills to be learned may take many weeks or even months to master.

11. Enjoy the self-exploration and growth. Do it with an attitude of childlike play, with thoughts such as "I wonder what I'll experience next." We are not static. Remember, each experience is different because we are continuously changing. It is only in death that change no longer occurs. Hence, offer yourself the richness of exploring the uncharted future.

12. Explore the Recommended Readings at the end of each chapter for more detailed presentations of the concepts.

Specific Instructions

Because the practices build upon the previous ones, the mastery of the earlier practices will enhance and deepen the later ones. Begin by scanning the workbook chapters: Introduction, Dynamic Relaxation, Cognitive Balance, and Self-Healing Through Imagery and Behavior Change. Notice that each chapter contains one or more practices, which are usually introduced by some background material. Each practice includes specific instructions, such as a guided script, and for each for each there are worksheets for you to complete: daily logs, weekly questions about your logs, and questions for group discussion and conclusions. We have found that participants increase their benefit if they share their experiences with others who are also doing the exercises.

We recommend that you

1. Record your experiences on the **log sheet** each day after practice. At the end of the week's practice, review your logs and answer the **questions**. If you are practicing these exercises with others, meet weekly and complete the **discussion and conclusions worksheet**.
2. Develop reminders to practice the mini-exercises during the day. It is through these mini-practices that awareness is fostered.

3. Remember that your experiences change. Each time you do a practice you are different; therefore, do not expect the same experience. Progress is not always slow and steady. There may be slumps and setbacks; there may also be big leaps ahead.
4. Act on your observations and insights; allow yourself to make mistakes. Mistakes offer us the opportunity to learn.

Some Precautions

Do not alter the use of your medications without consulting your health care provider. The following persons should proceed carefully and possibly receive guidance or supervision from a trained professional:

- Those who are taking medication such as sleeping pills, antihypertensive medication, tranquilizers, antidepressants, insulin, or thyroid supplement. These individuals should have their medications monitored—and altered, if necessary—during training.
- Those who have suffered traumatic or consciousness-altering experiences such as automobile accidents, near drowning, rape, psychedelic drugs, and (sometimes) anesthesia. These persons often need support in feeling and discharging emotions associated with these experiences; they may also find relaxation difficult.
- Persons with other psychological conditions, such as dealing with the death of a loved one and experiencing depersonalization (loss of identity) or "fugue" states (out of body experiences). Emotional support and close monitoring will be necessary.

It is further suggested that if illness is present, you should avoid focusing, during the beginning of training, on the area of concern. For example, an asthmatic may have difficulty focusing on breathing initially and should thus delay the breathing practice until the fifth or sixth practice session.

If uncomfortable feelings or experiences occur, in some cases you may need to adapt the practices, skip the section, and/or seek outside psychological/medical support. Frequently it will be possible to resume the practice after a few days' pause, since we all have an underlying drive toward health and integration.

If you generally block or suppress a need to cry or vomit, be aware that in deeply relaxed states occasionally such inhibitions are loosened and crying or vomiting may occur. This is normal.

APPROACHES TO SELF-REGULATION: OVERVIEW

With your eyes closed, imagine a lemon. Notice the deep yellow color, the two stubby ends, the sign "Sunkist" stamped on the side. Place the lemon on a cutting board and cut the lemon in half with your favorite kitchen knife. Notice the pressure in your hand as you cut. Feel the droplets of lemon juice sprinkling against your skin. Put the knife down and take one of the half lemons in your hand. Notice the droplets of lemon juice glistening in the light. Observe the half-cut seeds, the outer yellow rind, the pale yellow-white inner rind, the pulpy membranes containing the lemon juice. Now get a glass and squeeze the lemon so that the juice goes in the glass. Notice the tension in your hand and arm. Feel the droplets of lemon juice squirting against your skin. Hear the plopping of the seeds and pulp. Smell the pungent, sharp, tart odor. After having squeezed this half, take the other lemon half and squeeze the juice out of it into the glass. . . . Then put that lemon half down, and take the glass in your hand. Feel the coolness of the glass. Bring the glass to your lips, tilt the glass. Notice the pressure and coolness on the lower lip. Now taste and swallow the lemon juice. Observe the pulp and seeds as you swallow. (Peper and Williams, 1981, pp. 187–188)

As you read those words, perhaps you had a direct experience of salivating, swallowing, and puckering your lips. Observe how images and thoughts produced real physiologic responses in the body! We are equally capable of getting physically upset and distraught over an imagined event or worry that may never really happen. These are both examples of how the mind and body are not at all separate; in fact, any event in the mind is accompanied by a response in the body and vice versa. We are also very much affected by the environment in which we exist: the family and social environment; the quality of the air, water, and food we take in; our work or school situation; and, of course, our perceptions and feelings about all of these.

Rationale for Learning Relaxation

The rate of change in our society is constantly increasing, bringing greater pressures in many areas of life. We learn to work harder and to juggle multiple roles (such as career, family, and school). These pressures and stressors, including major crises and minor hassles, can lead to a breakdown in health. Indeed, up to 80% of today's health problems in America are considered to be linked to stress. When our health breaks down, we often seem to be at the mercy of an impersonal medical system in which we feel helpless and alienated.

People who are chronically stressed are placing an extra load on their bodies. The body has a limited amount of energy to be used for adaptation and change; conserving and regenerating it through relaxation practices is important for health and well-being. Conversely, when we become sick, we draw on our reserves and can easily get into "deficit spending." Rebuilding the energy reservoir can take time. Think about what happens in a prolonged drought. A single downpour does little to moisten the parched soil and may simply wash off with little beneficial effect. On the other hand, a slow trickle of rain over a long time will gradually restore the soil's moisture. Similarly, a single vacation in Hawaii may do little to build up the depleted energy reserves drained by prolonged stress and/or illness; a daily relaxation practice carried out over a few weeks or months may be much more restorative.

The body's alarm state, or "fight or flight" response, involves dramatic changes when a threat is perceived: The pituitary gland triggers the adrenals to secrete adrenaline, cortisol, and other hormones; heart rate and blood pressure increase; muscles tense in anticipation of running or fighting; blood leaves the skin in order to supply the muscles; digestion stops. This response can be life saving when the threat is physical; in modern life, however, it is frequently life *threatening*, when it is chronically reactivated without the opportunity for discharge through vigorous physical activity or deep relaxation. When stress is chronic, the body adapts (temporarily) and channels the strain into one or more organ systems. However, ultimately exhaustion ensues, these systems begin to break down, and the person becomes vulnerable to illness (Cannon, 1939; Selye, 1956, 1974). Sometimes it is possible to diminish stressors through prioritizing tasks, resolving conflicts, being more assertive, and so on. Even when you are unable to remove the sources of stress in your life, you can begin to reduce the toll stress takes on your body and to recharge your energy reservoirs by learning and using an effective relaxation technique.

Who Can Benefit?

Those who are suffering from the effects of excess physical and/or mental stress and tension, who are motivated to help heal themselves, and who have a desire for greater self-awareness can benefit by using this workbook.

There is more and more evidence of the importance of stress and attitude as codetermining factors in many illnesses and conditions, such as heart disease, cancer, arthritis, diabetes, hypertension, ulcers, colitis, asthma, allergies, premature aging, depression, eczema, headaches, back pain, insomnia, menstrual irregularities, infertility, increased susceptibility to infections, immune system disorders, and reduced performance (Justice, 1988; Levy, 1985; McEwen, 1990; Pelletier, 1977). In addition, many people who are in relatively good health still suffer from excess fatigue, anxiety, and muscle tension. Our mental and physical states are inextricably intertwined, so an integrated approach must include strategies for both mental and physical relaxation. Thus, even if you believe your problem areas are strictly psychological or interpersonal in origin, use of physical relaxation exercises can be highly beneficial. And even if you believe your condition has a strictly physical origin, cognitive and psychological approaches may be useful as well.

Other benefits may include improved sleep, enhanced awareness of the body, ability to regenerate one's energies quickly, increased concentration, and improvement in athletics, schoolwork, or any performance task. There may be a decrease in emotional reactivity and a concurrent sense of inner peace and integration. Sometimes the benefits are quite unexpected. For example, one woman with panic attacks, who said she had never relaxed in her life before learning dynamic relaxation, finally learned to lower her shoulders. As a result, she reported, "I had to readjust my bra straps!"

Types of Relaxation

Deep Relaxation. Many people believe that relaxation consists of watching TV, socializing with friends, or listening to music. While these may be pleasant, there is a difference between such activities and the ability to achieve deep-muscle relaxation, which allows for renewal of vital bodily processes and healing. When the muscles are profoundly relaxed, a rebalancing takes place. Heart rate, blood pressure, breathing, digestion, and metabolism return to a normal state; the immune system's healing abilities are enhanced; and repair and restoration take place (see Chapter 2). Breath, which is under both conscious and unconscious control, is a very basic aspect of relaxation. In learning self-regulation of our breathing, we can begin to "switch off" the fight-or-flight response. Slow, deep diaphragmatic breathing is life affirming and restorative. In this breathing pattern the diameter of the abdomen expands during inhalation and decreases during exhalation. Such a pattern usually occurs when one is at peace and relaxed. It not only brings in more oxygen, enabling clearer thinking, but it also lowers the sympathetic nervous system arousal, which is responsible for tight muscles, racing heart, high blood pressure, and feelings of anxiety. Since it is under conscious control, we can always choose to take a few quieting breaths in order to initiate a relaxation process or ease feelings of fear or anger (see "Breathing: The Mind–Body Bridge: Practice 3" in Chapter 2).

Differential Relaxation. Through this workbook you can learn the skills of differential relaxation, or the letting go of muscles not needed for a particular task. For example, while driving many people unconsciously tense their jaw and shoulder muscles, which are not needed to drive a car effectively. Such wasted muscle effort, known as *dysponesis*, needlessly drains off our energy reserves (Whatmore & Kohli, 1974). Systematic practice of dynamic relaxation methods increases your awareness of whether your muscles are tense or relaxed as you go about your daily activities, thus giving you the choice of releasing unnecessary tension. *Awareness gives you choices!* Then you can save that adaptation energy, which would have been wasted on unnecessary muscle tension, for other activities—such as self-healing (see "Reducing Tension/Increasing Awareness: Practice 5" in Chapter 2).

Generalized Relaxation. When a skill is practiced over and over, in a variety of situations, it becomes "overlearned" or automatic; very little conscious awareness is needed to produce the behavior. Also, we can condition certain responses at will. Certain cues in our environment produce automatic responses which can be useful; for example, at a red light or stop sign, we step on the brake almost without thinking about it. Similarly, we can condition ourselves to relax certain muscles, or to breathe slowly and deeply, in response to a cue such as the words *relax, calm,* or *serene*. Or we can invoke a relaxing, reassuring image; a small object such as a seashell on the desk or in the pocket can be a reminder of a calmer time (see "Developing a Personal Relaxation Image: Practice 4" in Chapter 2). A cue for relaxation can be anything we choose. With practice we can even train ourselves to let a red light or a ringing telephone become a cue to relax. For example, when the phone rings, you may habitually tighten your shoulders; instead, you now choose to use the phone ringing as a signal to relax your shoulders and breathe before answering it (see "Quick and Warm and Generalizing Relaxation: Practices 6 and 7" in Chapter 2). Systematic practice of relaxation teaches our muscles that tension is no longer the norm; we have the choice of relaxing, and relaxing can become the new habit instead of tension.

Deep Relaxation as a Gateway to the Unconscious.   As restorative as it is all by itself, deep relaxation has still other benefits. When the muscles are quiet, the conscious rational mind also quiets, allowing access to intuition. The highly verbal, analytical, judgmental part of the mind is also sometimes referred to as the left brain. The right brain is intuitive, visual, and synthetic and thinks in pictures or images, perceives relationships and wholes, and is more in touch with the emotions. Most of the time we are not paying attention to the quiet messages from our right brain because the left brain is busy censoring them! Deep relaxation can temporarily get the left brain out of the way and allow right-brain inputs. Thus, relaxation can be helpful in interrupting habitual negative thought patterns and opening the mind to new possibilities. Greater creativity and problem-solving abilities may emerge spontaneously (Green and Green, 1977). Valuable messages about changes we need to make for our greater health and well-being often arise.

Cognitive Stress Management

The events in our lives can be perceived not as inherently good or bad but as neutral. It's how we choose to view the events that determines, in large part, how we respond—with helplessness, hopelessness, optimism, or humor. If we use language which implies that we're helpless victims, then that view of our world is strengthened; the opposite is also true. Some of our language use is habitual and outside of our conscious awareness. Our inner dialogue may include not only words but also pictures, gut feelings, premonitions, and expectations. A person who was abused as a child may have learned a sense of helplessness that extends into adult life, including situations where, in reality, the adult has choices and need not be powerless. The good news is that unrealistic assessments of ourselves and the world (based on past experience) can be revised and changed. Changing language to emphasize our choices and capabilities is a step in that direction (see "Changing the Internal Dialogue: Practice 9" in Chapter 3).

A key aspect of coping with stress, as described in the serenity prayer, is to recognize which things we can control and which we can't and then act appropriately or let go:

> God grant me the serenity
> To accept the things I cannot change,
> Courage to change the things I can and
> Wisdom to know the difference.

A major cognitive coping process is *reframing*. This is learning to redefine threats as challenges or opportunities and can be very empowering. Look, for example, at the difference between calling a woman "preorgasmic" and calling her "frigid." The second term implies a hopeless and negative situation while the first implies a situation that can develop and change and is full of potential. Reframing threats as opportunities can mean an increased willingness to see even an illness or symptom as meeting a need (which may have been unacknowledged) and can direct us to make a change in our lifestyle. Mental rehearsal, in which we imagine the steps needed for success instead of reliving our failures, is an important tool for overcoming problems and encouraging behavior changes (see "Transforming Failure into Success: Practice 10" in Chapter 3).

Another cognitive coping process that encourages self-acceptance and integration is to write about past traumas (see Practice 11, "Freeing the Hidden Secrets" in Chapter 3). With this new awareness we can make changes and find new ways to get our needs met, thus removing the need for the illness or symptom (see "Converting the Advantages of Illness: Practice 12" in Chapter 3).

Self-Healing Through Imagery and Behavior Change

There is increasing recognition of the power of mental imagery to promote self-healing of diseases. Carl Simonton pioneered this work with cancer patients, and Martin Rossman and David Bresler have reported positive results with people having a wide variety of afflictions, often after little or no progress using traditional "allopathic" (Western medical) approaches (Rossman, 1987; Simonton, Matthews-Simonton, & Creighton, 1978).

Imagery exercises may take several forms. To begin with, it is useful to practice the previously acquired relaxation skills to allow a free flow of spontaneous imagery. These messages from the right brain may provide valuable information about the nature of a symptom or illness, as well as clues for action steps to help relieve it. For example, a man seeking to heal himself of obesity and overeating received images of himself as a child feeling unloved and insecure and eating to fill the void he felt inside. This led him to the awareness that dieting alone would probably not work; he needed to find ways to obtain nurturance other than by eating.

In imagery practice, first imagine the problem area or area of concern; then imagine the healing process taking place. Finally, imagine yourself whole, healed, filled with energy and living life without the problem. Often it is helpful to make a drawing of each image so that it may be viewed from a different perspective, one that may offer a clearer illustration of the illness and healing process.

Not all imagery is visual in nature. Athletes practice mental imagery using multisensory approaches. For example, a basketball player may imagine the feeling of the ball in his or her hands while dribbling around the court, the sensation in the legs while leaping into the air, the sound of the ball smoothly landing in the net. The more senses you can bring to bear, the more successful (and fun!) your practice is likely to be. A number of research studies have demonstrated that imagined practice improves performance and accuracy. Mental rehearsal may have a wide variety of applications for changing behavior as well as for healing. Yet another step in successful imagery practice is finding ways to associate imagery with various daily routines. A woman with acne created a face-washing ritual that involved visualizing caves with bits of green scum in them (like an enlarged photo of facial pores harboring bacteria); she visualized the ocean washing through these caves and removing all the scum as she washed her face with warm water several times daily.

Do you remember a time when the loss of a love or another depressing event was in the back of your mind for a period of time? Without conscious thought, that underlying awareness colored your daily experiences. Worrying (negative mental rehearsal) is another example; an image, a word, or a feeling is in the background over a period of time. Successful imagers develop a background awareness of their healing image that is everpresent. Just as we learn to take mini-breaks for relaxation throughout the day, triggered by cues, so too can we learn to do mini-practices of imagery cued to everyday events such as face-washing, drinking a glass of water, walking, urinating, and so forth.

Behavior change often follows naturally from exploring imagery. For example, a person seeking to heal a condition of low energy and depression may receive an image of herself or himself hiking or dancing. It is very important to act upon the insights gained from imagery (in this case, to make specific plans to hike or dance) as soon as possible.

Undertaking behavior change with a sense of excitement, challenge, and support (rather than thinking, "I should," "I ought to," or "I can't") is much more likely when you follow a well-planned strategy. Such a strategy will incorporate setting achievable goals and objectives, choosing positive self-talk, collecting data on your present behavior, manipulating the cues in your environment, rewarding yourself, arranging social support, using mental rehearsal for troubleshooting, keeping records of your progress, and making adaptations as you go.

LOGGING YOUR RESPONSES TO STRESS: PRACTICE 1

When you take time to give attention to yourself, you may be surprised to find out things you do not know about yourself, and especially surprised when you find what you thought you knew was not quite right at all.

PARTICIPANT

Before beginning the journey of self-change through dynamic relaxation, images, and thoughts, take some time to observe your present patterns of responding to stress. This is a way of taking your bearings and discovering what your *baseline* is, the starting point from which you will measure your progress.

We are all confronted with many stressors in our busy and hectic lives. There are minor and major hassles that occur day after day and add up to a large stress load; there are stressful life events and changes, both positive and negative, that force us to adapt. There are job and interpersonal and home stressors. How aware are you of both the stressors and your responses to them? Our responses to stress include our physical and emotional reactions, what we say to ourselves, and what we do. These responses may be more damaging to us than we realize. They have been learned over time and are often habitual. If these habits are not helpful to us, they can also be unlearned.

Use the stress log for at least 2 days; a week is preferable. This will help you develop awareness and build motivation for change. Some participants found that keeping a stress log gave them insight into ways to resolve chronic, predictable stressors; others noted an increased awareness of how negative and critical their thoughts and self-talk are.

A major component of this workbook is to learn new, less destructive patterns for coping with stress. During this self-monitoring period, whenever you are aware of a strong emotional reaction *or* whenever you notice some of the indicators of your body's stress response (such as muscle tension, shallow breathing, tight stomach, racing heart), get out your pen or pencil and jot down some notes. What was the event, the associated emotions, your thoughts, and your physical response? What did you do? Describe it on the **Log Sheet: Practice 1**. At the end of the monitoring period, answer **Questions: Practice 1**. Then meet with your group and complete **Discussion and Conclusions: Practice 1**.

Name _____ Date _____

Log Sheet   Responses to Stress: Practice 1

Whenever you feel stressed, write down the following: the stressful event/situation, the associated emotions, thoughts, action and physical responses/reactions. Use more pages if you like.

Stressful event	Emotions	Thoughts (self-talk)	Action	Physical response
Example:				
Getting lost	Frustrated and angry	I am so stupid I'll be late.	Continued to drive without asking for directions	Fight your Sweaty palms

Stressful event	Emotions	Thoughts (self-talk)	Action	Physical response
_____	_____	_____	_____	_____
_____	_____	_____	_____	_____
_____	_____	_____	_____	_____
_____	_____	_____	_____	_____
_____	_____	_____	_____	_____
_____	_____	_____	_____	_____
_____	_____	_____	_____	_____
_____	_____	_____	_____	_____
_____	_____	_____	_____	_____
_____	_____	_____	_____	_____
_____	_____	_____	_____	_____
_____	_____	_____	_____	_____
_____	_____	_____	_____	_____
_____	_____	_____	_____	_____
_____	_____	_____	_____	_____
_____	_____	_____	_____	_____
_____	_____	_____	_____	_____
_____	_____	_____	_____	_____
_____	_____	_____	_____	_____
_____	_____	_____	_____	_____
_____	_____	_____	_____	_____
_____	_____	_____	_____	_____
_____	_____	_____	_____	_____
_____	_____	_____	_____	_____
_____	_____	_____	_____	_____
_____	_____	_____	_____	_____
_____	_____	_____	_____	_____
_____	_____	_____	_____	_____
_____	_____	_____	_____	_____
_____	_____	_____	_____	_____
_____	_____	_____	_____	_____
_____	_____	_____	_____	_____
_____	_____	_____	_____	_____
_____	_____	_____	_____	_____
_____	_____	_____	_____	_____
_____	_____	_____	_____	_____
_____	_____	_____	_____	_____
_____	_____	_____	_____	_____
_____	_____	_____	_____	_____
_____	_____	_____	_____	_____
_____	_____	_____	_____	_____

Name _____ Date _____

Questions   Responses to Stress: Practice 1

1. Were the stressful events/situations you experienced within or outside your control? Were these routine or unexpected?

_____

_____

_____

2. What emotions were evoked by the stressors?

_____

_____

_____

3. How did your thoughts or self-talk make the situation better or worse?

_____

_____

_____

4. How did your actions influence the situations?

_____

_____

_____

5. What physical responses to stress did you notice in your body?

_____

_____

_____

6. Did your body respond similarly or differently to different stressors?

_____

_____

_____

7. Other observations: _____

_____

_____

Responses and Conclusions Responses to Stress: Practice 1

1. What stressors did group members share in common?

_____

_____

_____

2. Among group members, what effect did monitoring of stress response have on the experience of the event?

_____

_____

_____

_____

3. How did group members think and act under stress? What were the similarities and differences?

_____

_____

_____

_____

4. What similarities and differences were there in physical/emotional responses to stress?

_____

_____

_____

_____

5. Topics for which instructor consultation would be helpful:

_____

_____

_____

List your group members: _____ _____

_____ _____ _____

_____ _____ _____

IMPORTANT VARIABLES TO OPTIMIZE TRAINING[3]

In order to learn unstressing techniques, you need to optimize the conditions under which you may relax. These conditions involve the reduction of stimuli impinging upon you, both physical/environmental and psychological/internal. You can also adopt behaviors that encourage success.

Physical Variables

1. Select an environment where the following conditions are met:
    A. Training, once begun, will not be interrupted. (Unplug the phone, put a note on the outside of the door, inform others that you are going to begin training, etc.) It may be important to explain what you are doing to your family, housemates, or significant others. Enlist their support. With young children, you may need to time your relaxation during their naps.
    B. Noise is minimal. (Don't begin training next to the TV or recreation room.)
    C. The lighting is subdued, not harsh or glaring.
    D. The temperature is comfortable (a cold room makes it difficult to relax, an overly warm room may induce sleepiness).
    E. The chair, bed, or carpet on which training is done is comfortable and provides good support.
2. Choose the position for training that is most comfortable for you—either lying down or sitting.
    A. If lying down, you may want to place a pillow underneath your head so your neck and shoulders are comfortable. Place a pillow underneath your knees so that your lower back is not strained. Be sure the surface beneath is comfortable (use carpet or foam). Make sure your legs are not crossed and that your toes are pointing outward. Keep your arms at your side and not touching your trunk. (If you tend to fall asleep very easily or are very tired when doing these practices, you will probably do better in a sitting position.)
    B. If sitting, make sure the chair offers sufficient support so that you do not fall over when you relax. Make sure the height of the chair is such that your feet are flat on the floor and that there is not undue pressure on your thighs (if the chair is too high, place a telephone book or stool under your feet). Sit with your legs and feet uncrossed and with thighs relaxed so that your legs are slightly separated. Let your arms rest on the arms of the chair or rest them gently in your lap. Let your head either hang forward or be supported by the back of the chair. Be sure your neck is not strained. A recliner is great.
3. Scan your body and check if there is anything impinging upon and/or constricting it; if so, loosen or remove the constricting or impinging items.
    A. Often we become unaware of the constricting nature of our clothing. For

example, when you first put on your shoes in the morning, you may feel the shoe enclosing your foot, yet after a few minutes you are unaware of the shoe. When you scan (i.e., feel what is going on inside) your body and attention is brought to your foot, you again become aware of the shoe. During relaxation, we often become aware of the constricting sensation and are distracted from the process of relaxation. Check for such items as shoes, a tight collar, tie, wig, glasses, contact lenses, socks with elastic tops, hair barrette or rubber band, watch, ring, heavy pendant, wallet or keys in pocket, belt, bra, and girdle. If you are working in a group and are uncomfortable about loosening personal items, go through the exercise as best you can and next time you practice make sure to dress so that these items are not a problem.

B. Items that appear comfortable in our normal posture may physically prevent the process of relaxation. For example, jeans that are tight across the abdomen prevent the letting go and expansion of the abdominal wall. They force thoracic breathing and prevent the more relaxing diaphragmatic breathing. Check for such items as belt, tight pants, panty hose, or tight corset.

C. An item that appears comfortable in our normal posture may demand bracing while we relax. For example, if you are wearing glasses and your head tilts forward during relaxation, you may tend to tighten your neck muscles to prevent your head from nodding and your glasses from falling. Similarly, a woman with a short skirt may hold her knees together and not let her legs relax, and people with dentures may tighten their jaw because of the fear that the dentures may fall out.

D. A physical state may also distract us from relaxing. For example, having a full bladder or being either very hungry or full may make it difficult to relax. Being extremely tired may either cause sleepiness and mind wandering or a state of feeling keyed-up. Avoid caffeine for at least 2 hours prior to relaxation.

Psychological Variables

There are certain attitudes of the trainee that encourage relaxation. These include the following:

1. *Passive attention.* This is an attitude of nonstriving—of allowing versus forcing or trying—and is characterized by the absence of concern for performance and end result.

2. *Nonjudgmental acceptance.* This attitude includes not explaining, interpreting, or labeling an experience as good or bad but letting it be and describing it without judgment. It implies not comparing one experience to another but, rather, experiencing each new situation afresh (watch out for words like *because,* and *should* and for expressions like *the reason is*). Also, if thoughts and feelings arise, instead of pushing them away, gently accept them and release them.

3. *Mindfulness.* This is an attitude of remaining present, watchful, and aware of what is happening without becoming involved or captured by the images or feelings. Being truly present implies the absence of anticipating, ruminating, or mind wandering.

Behavioral Variables

There are a number of strategies that facilitate home practice and generalization of relaxation skills. The following are a few suggestions:

1. Keep log notes. As previously mentioned, these notes concerning your experience, time of day, mood before and after the practice will provide valuable data to help you choose the best times and settings. Notice situations when it is easy and when it is more difficult for you to practice. This enables you to select those situations that encourage practice. For example, you may find that you practice a relaxation skill with another person more often than by yourself; if so, structure your practice time with a friend or fellow classmate. Also, some participants have reported that looking over their log notes reinspired them.
2. Schedule a regular practice time and associate it with an existing behavior. For example, you may practice after watching the evening news or before dinner. It is preferable not to practice too soon after a large meal. If you tend to fall asleep easily, it is best not to practice late in the evening. It is also best initially not to tie relaxing with going to sleep.
3. Give yourself a reinforcer meaningful to you when you practice. For example, if you practice for a week, treat yourself to a movie or special meal (Thorenson & Mahoney, 1974; Watson & Tharp, 1981).

PERSONALIZING YOUR EXPERIENCE

Making Your Own Tapes[4]

I was not used to hearing gentle, pleasant, encouraging words from myself.
                                                                    PARTICIPANT

For each of the relaxation practices there is a script, which is designed to be read aloud and taped by the trainee. There are many benefits involved in making your own relaxation tapes. The extra time required can be well worth it. Making your own tapes gives you the ability to tailor a relaxation sequence to your own needs. For example, if you have lower back pain, you might choose to eliminate or change those instructions that might affect your back. If you typically do the practice before starting a work period, you might want to conclude the tape with a suggestion that you are now awake, alert, and mentally focused. If you have trouble relaxing a particular part of your body, you might decide to repeat the tensing and relaxing instructions an extra time for that area. You may want to tape the instructions with your favorite music playing softly in the background. When you make the tape with your personal relaxation imagery, in Practice 4, you can provide background sounds such as ocean waves, birds singing, and so forth. Certain words may have more pleasant associations for you than those in the scripts, and you can substitute them. For example, some people initially respond negatively to the word *relax* because of having been told impatiently, "Would you relax!!"

If English is your second language, deep relaxation may be more successful if you translate all the scripts into your native language.

Relaxation is not different from self-acceptance. Listening to your own voice telling you to relax helps you to internalize the instructions and promotes self-acceptance. Many people who began by disliking the sound of their voice on tape ended by enjoying listening to themselves. One woman said that making her own tape, with the appropriate pauses, helped her learn to listen more in dialogue with other people and to slow down the pace of her hectic life.

Here are some helpful hints for making your tapes:

1. Before making your tape, practice reading the script aloud, if possible to a friend or family member, to get feedback on your pacing. As you make the tape, imagine doing the practice or actually do it (or lead another person through it). This will help your pacing.
2. Make the tape at a time when you're not feeling rushed so that your voice will convey relaxation. Be sure to speak slowly and breathe diaphragmatically throughout. Allow your voice to drop to a slightly lower pitch than you use in everyday speech.
3. Allow plenty of time for the relaxation phase after muscle tensing. A good rule is to allow 7 to 10 seconds for tensing and 15 to 30 seconds for relaxation. Whenever the script indicates . . . , pause for a few seconds. Most people tend not to allow enough time for relaxation. Quiet space on the tape is OK.

Like the first pancake, the first attempt at making a tape is not always successful. Think of your first one as an experiment, and if need be, do it over. It will be a good learning experience!

Development of a Personal Ritual for Relaxation

A wonderful fact about the mind is that our responses can be conditioned. Just as we learn to associate certain cues (e.g., a ringing phone or the sight of an angry person) with tension, so too can we learn to associate certain cues with relaxation. As soon as we encounter a relaxation cue, we begin to release tension almost automatically. This can work for you to help deepen your relaxation practices and to allow you to begin relaxing more quickly. The following are some examples of rituals and cues:

- Putting on comfortable, loose sweatpants
- Getting into your favorite chair

- Lighting a candle or a stick of incense
- Ringing a meditation bell or bowl
- Taking three slow, deep breaths
- Putting on some quiet, soothing background music
- Putting a favorite stuffed animal, blanket, or other comforting item nearby (see Pavlov Exercise in Chapter 2 for ideas)

When you are beginning your relaxation practice, it sometimes helps to use a checklist so that important items are not forgotten (see checklist in Chapter 2).

Why Keep Log Notes?

Writing is an important way of bringing language to our experiences, which helps us to understand, assimilate, and integrate what has happened. Writing brings the amorphous into a concrete form and gives it a sense of containment. It allows us to transport the subtle, evanescent, and easily forgotten inner experience into our everyday consciousness, thus providing the bridge between insight and action. Later, the written words make it possible to look back and reflect upon patterns in our experience that would otherwise not be knowable because so much of our behavior and responses occur automatically.

Another important function of writing is the cultivation of that part of the mind that is the "witness," the part that observes, with calm detachment, everything that we experience. This form of awareness is also developed through meditation. Such awareness can be very valuable in aiding behavior changes. For example, one can simply observe a desire to run away from a frightening stimulus, without giving in to it. Or one can observe, perhaps many times in an hour, a desire or craving for, say, alcohol or sugar, again without having to act on it. Thus, we come to know ourselves and to create greater freedom from old habit patterns. Journal keeping is transformative.

Reflection and Integration: Summarizing Your Experiences

Looking over my logs and questions over the last four weeks, I could really notice the improvement. The emotions which were hidden for so long finally came to the surface. I could feel them and accept them for what they were. I was mindful and realized that these are patterns I have repeated for many years. With distance, I could accept and notice movement and change. I finally know that I am growing.

Looking back over the previous weeks' experience offers a possibility of integration, acceptance, and growth. We recommend highly that after every major chapter of this workbook, you look back over your comments in the logs and discussion pages. Looking back allows you to organize your experience. As you review the previous weeks' experiences, you may note that significant changes have occurred. These can include increased awareness of more subtle cues of tension; recognition of helpful and destructive life patterns; reduction or disappearance of symptoms such as tension headaches, migraine, or insomnia; and even an enhanced appreciation of the remarkable self-healing potential intrinsic in each of us.

Instructions for Writing a Summary Paper. After having practiced a series of the exercises, write a summary paper (three to five pages) about your experiences. Write these papers after Dynamic Relaxation (Practice 8); Cognitive Balance (Practice 12), and Self-Healing Through Imagery and Behavior Change (Practice 14). Reflect back over the previous practices by rereading your Log sheets, Question sheets, and Discussion and Conclusions sheets. In these papers address some of the following concerns:

1. What was your experience with the different practices?
2. How did each practice deepen different components of your self?
3. What benefits did you observe as a result?
4. What common patterns underlay your experiences?
5. What difficulties or challenges did you encounter, and how did you cope with them?
6. In what ways were the small group discussions helpful?
7. What have you learned about yourself through the practice of these techniques?
8. If you could do it over again (repeat the practices), what would you do differently?
9. What have you learned that you will apply to the next practice?

SUGGESTED READINGS

Bailey, C. (1991). *The New Fit or Fat.* Boston: Houghton Mifflin.

Chopra, D. (1989). *Quantum Healing.* New York: Bantam.

Cousins, N. (1989). *Head First: The Biology of Hope.* New York: Dutton.

Dossey, L. (1989). *Recovering the Soul.* New York: Bantam.

Davis, M., Eshelman, E. R., and McKay, M. (1982). *The Relaxation and Stress Reduction Workbook.* Oakland, CA: New Harbinger.

Frank, A. W. (1991). *At the Will of the Body.* Boston: Houghton Mifflin.

Girdano, D. A., Everly, G. S., & Dusek, D. E. (1990). *Controlling Stress and Tension: A Holistic Approach.* Englewood Cliffs, NJ: Prentice-Hall.

Kunz, D. (1985). *Spiritual Aspects of the Healing Arts.* Wheaton, IL: Quest Books.

Ornish, D. (1990). *Dr. Dean Ornish's Program for Reversing Heart Disease.* New York: Random House.

Payer, L. (1988). *Medicine and Culture.* New York: Penguin Books.

Robbins, J. (1987). *Diet for a New America.* Walpole, NH: Still-point.

Sagan, L. A. (1987). *The Health of Nations: True Causes of Sickness and Well-Being.* New York: Basic Books.

Siegel, B. S. (1989). *Peace, Love and Healing.* New York: Harper & Row.

Chapter 2
Dynamic Relaxation

The bow too tensely strung is easily broken.
PUBLILIUS SYRUS

Human beings, once they advance from crawling on all fours to walking on two, no longer need regress to a limping posture once they become older. That is to say, the bodily decrepitude presumed under the myth of aging is not inevitable. It is, by and large, both avoidable and reversible.
THOMAS HANNA

INTRODUCTION TO DYNAMIC RELAXATION

The first awareness is of how much we abuse our bodies. Then comes compassion, then behavior change. Compassion and gentleness are healing.

Edmund Jacobson (1970, 1974) introduced progressive relaxation, a graded series of muscle tensing and releasing exercises for the learning of profound muscular and mental relaxation (Bernstein & Borkovec, 1973). Jacobson's premise was that by voluntarily relaxing the muscles we can, in fact, slow down the activity of the sympathetic nervous system, which is responsible for the fight-or-flight response and nervous tension. When the sympathetic nervous system is quiet, the parasympathetic becomes more dominant, allowing the heart rate and blood pressure to go down, blood vessels to dilate, the internal organs to relax, and restorative body processes to take place. "If you relax your skeletal muscles sufficiently (those over which you have control), the internal muscles tend to relax likewise.... Excessive tension ... in the visceral muscles depends more or less upon the presence of excessive tension in the skeletal muscles" (Jacobson, 1976, p. 158). Thus, control over processes that we tend to think of as involuntary, such as pulse rate and blood pressure, becomes possible.

Overfatigued and nervous people lose the natural ability to relax and, in fact, do not know which muscles are tense. With practice, this can be relearned. The goal at first is to learn how to relax so deeply that even residual tension is gone. When residual tension has been relaxed away, "mental and emotional activity dwindle or disappear for brief periods" (Jacobson, 1976, p. 155). The exercises then progress gradually from the ability to achieve deep relaxation voluntarily while lying down or sitting comfortably to the ability to recognize and eliminate unnecessary muscle tension during everyday activities. Ultimately, relaxation becomes a more habitual state than tension.

Since it was first introduced, many modifications have been made to Jacobson's technique. The original method called for a week of daily practice in relaxing each muscle group (e.g., the right wrist). Our modification of Jacobson's exercises, which we call dynamic relaxation,[1] includes a larger number of muscle groups and incorporates some breathing and visualization techniques as well as the tensing and relaxing.

The scripts in this section guide you through the steps for learning dynamic relaxation and diaphragmatic breathing. Each script is to be practiced once each day for a week. You may either memorize these scripts, have a friend guide you through them, or tape-record the scripts and play them back during your practice. After each daily practice, note your experiences on the appropriate **Log Sheet**, and at the end of each week, review your experiences and answer the **Questions**. Then meet with your group and complete the **Discussion and Conclusions** sheet.

In learning dynamic relaxation, it is helpful to have a skilled trainer guide you through the scripts for the first time. A trainer may also lead the group discussion, scan log sheets, and observe participants during sessions for unusual physiological or psychological reactions. If you are learning these scripts on your own, monitor yourself for unusual reactions and see the section "Some Precautions" in Chapter 1. Go through the following exercise to experience the basic processes, tensing and letting go, involved in dynamic relaxation:

> Choose a comfortable position. Close your eyes. Bend your hand back at the wrist with your fingers pointing upward. Hold this position for 5 to 10 seconds. Check that you are not tightening any other part of your body; check your shoulders and jaw.[2] Are you breathing comfortably? Bring your attention to your forearm. Observe the sensations of tightening. What are they? Mentally describe the sensations in the present tense without judgment. If your attention drifts away, bring it back to your forearm. All at once, completely release the tension that holds your fingers and hand upright. Let gravity pull your hand down; do not actively put it down. Let your hand and arm relax for at least 20 seconds. Relaxing is not doing. Observe the sensations of relaxation (letting go). What are they? How do they differ from those of tightening? If you did not feel any sensations, hold the muscle tight until you feel something, such as pain or discomfort. If you find it difficult to let go, try the exercise after a sauna, hot tub, or a massage.

SUGGESTIONS FOR GETTING STARTED ON RELAXATION EXERCISES

These helpful hints have been offered by previous participants.

- If possible, approach the exercises without expectations—just curiosity.
- View the practice time as a reward or "time out for me," not a task. Don't push yourself to do it "right." Let go of performance issues.
- If you are having trouble with a portion of the exercise, modify or leave out that part.
- At first, try varying the time and place and setting to find what works best for you; try doing it away from home, too. Experiment! After you discover what works well, stay with a standard time and place so that you form a positive habit.
- To get into the right mood, begin by recalling a memory of a pleasant experience.
- The hardest part may be setting aside 20 to 30 minutes a day for yourself. Remember, you're worth it! You're forming a new, life-enhancing habit. If your mind wanders, visualize each part of the body relaxing as you do the exercises; and be very aware of internal feelings as well. Especially, visualize and feel the lungs expanding and contracting with each breath. If motivation is a problem, give yourself little rewards just for doing the practice each week.
- Anticipate possible problems doing relaxation at home or at work. Then develop an alternative plan.
- If you dislike working with tapes, memorize the script instead. This will be handy in helping you to generalize the skills later.
- To help set the mood, you might want to listen to soft music (classical or new age); then, later the music will be a conditioned cue for relaxation.
- Have a confidant, or buddy, to share your relaxation experiences with. Be sure to make use of the people in your discussion group. Your input may help someone else and, similarly, you may find solutions and reassurance. Remember practicing relaxation exercises is a new experience. Be gentle to yourself.
- Be aware of and acknowledge which part of your body holds the most chronic tension, and spend extra time with that part. Exhale through tight muscles.
- Tailor the end of the script for yourself: If you want a quick energy boost, give yourself some energizing suggestions; if you want to go to sleep soon, give yourself some quieting suggestions.
- You can enhance your relaxation by taking a hot bath before, during, or after the practice. Or start out with some gentle stretches or shake out your arms and legs.
- Make a note on the scripts of the parts you find helpful. You can use these parts to create your own script later on (Practice 8).

POSSIBLE PROBLEMS AND SOLUTIONS WHILE PRACTICING RELAXATION

Before commencing the practice, read through the following list of problems that commonly occur during practice and their suggested solutions. If you encounter any of the following problems, refer back to this section.

1. *Muscle cramps.* Stop tightening the muscle when you begin to sense pain or cramping; massage or move the cramped muscle while keeping rest of the body relaxed.
2. *Laughter or feeling self-conscious.* Practice in private, or just let feelings be and return attention to practice.
3. *Difficulty maintaining attention.* Describe changing sensations out loud during tension and relaxing; refocus your attention on the sensations.
4. *Ruminating over thoughts.* Write down your thoughts and concerns before you do the practices. By writing them down, you can be reassured that they will not be lost. Or, notice the thought and let it go.
5. *Sleepiness.* Do exercise at different time of day, get enough sleep, and practice while sitting up or for shorter periods of time.
6. *Experience of body parts changing, for example, becoming disassociated or increasing in size.* Allow experience to continue, as this indicates relaxation is occurring; if necessary, open eyes to check out body part.
7. *Uncomfortable emotion such as anger or sadness arising.* If the emotion is not too threatening, allow yourself to experience it without judgment. This is the body's way of releasing previously unconscious feelings that have been locked into the soma. Another strategy is to focus upon the breath in order to breathe through the emotion. Sharing the emotions that come up for you with others may also be helpful; often you will discover that you are not alone. If none of the above solutions work for you, you may also want to experiment with a shortened relaxation session, that is, do just half of a script at a given time.
8. *Family members don't understand or accept what you are doing, ridicule you, or bother you during the practice.* Do not keep your relaxation practices a secret from your family, thinking they won't understand. Explain to them, as best you can, what you are doing and why. Invite them to try it with you. Let them know of any positive benefits you are experiencing. Alleviate their fears (if any); some people feel threatened by new behavior in their loved ones and need reassurance that you haven't "gone off the deep end." Share the scientific data on relaxation as a means of stress reduction and health promotion.
9. *Overwhelming emotions, pain, frightening or excessive reactions.* Stop doing the exercise for a while, then resume with caution. Or seek professional consultation.

DYNAMIC RELAXATION: PRACTICE 2

Hardest Trust

Rumination carries on for precise seconds.
Then a tidal shift,
Mind anticipates for so many more:
A tangled compound worry of cause
to effects to a new cause for each and on.

Then try to trust.
"Let go," the three or four remembered voices
and two or three remembered pairs of hands
tell you all at once, then each in turn.
Let go, you feel then
Trust appears fleetingly of itself,
And then you try it out of itself again.

Rocking back and forth in and out of try,
Out of was, out of will be,
From each to the other, only glimpsing of now.

Trust, again building on itself from step to step,
Moves in and out gently
From back then to someday led by try.
And then, finally,
The balancing point.
Perfect, effortless, for this moment
That does not exist as a moment,
This is present as we don't recognize it—
This is peace.

LESLI FULLERTON

You may complete the Dynamic Relaxation exercises either lying down or sitting in a chair. If your position inhibits the tightening and letting go of a muscle group or if the directions do not feel quite appropriate or clear, modify the script to make it appropriate for you. Remember the following general points:

1. Keep your attention on the muscle group being tightened and relaxed.
2. Breathe easily and smoothly throughout.
3. Tighten only muscles that you are being directed to tighten, letting the rest of the body stay relaxed.
4. Have a confidant, or buddy, with whom to share and discuss your experiences of dynamic relaxation.
5. Complete your log notes immediately after your practice.
6. Keep a journal to record dreams or other significant insights as they come up.
7. Go over the Checklist for Relaxation Practice.

Each day, allot 20 to 30 minutes for the practice. This time period may be perceived as a "time-out" period during which the body and mind are allowed to relax and regenerate.

Checklist for Relaxation Practice

____ Phone unplugged (if possible)

____ Pet(s) out of the room

____ Note on door or family/roommate(s) informed

____ Lighting turned low/drapes pulled

____ Temperature adjusted for comfort

____ Appropriate pillows for knee support

____ Bladder emptied

____ Tape player and your self-recorded tape ready

____ Shoes removed

____ Clothing loosened (especially at neck and waist)

____ Jewelry, watch, glasses, etc., removed

____ Log sheet and pen ready to record before and after notes

____ Clock or watch within view

____ Assume an attitude of passive attention, "whatever happens."

Write in your personal ritual steps here:

_____

_____

_____

_____

_____

Dynamic Relaxation Script*

Begin by doing your personal ritual to initiate the shift toward relaxation . . . Remember, the important thing is not to be concerned about doing it "right"; just follow the instructions and observe with a gentle awareness what is going on in your body. Get into a comfortable position. Be sure your belt and pants are loose, your legs are uncrossed, your glasses and watch are off, and your shoulders are loose. If you wear hard contacts, you may want to remove them. Each time you are asked to tense your muscles, imagine that you are putting all your body tension into those muscles. When you are asked to relax, let go completely and immediately of all the tension. Focus your awareness on the sensations in your muscles.

*In the script, three dots (. . .) indicate a pause.

Close your eyes. Now clench your right fist . . . tighter and tighter . . . Continue to breathe slowly and deeply, from your belly, as you clench your fist . . . Allow your lips to be slightly parted; exhale through your mouth, whispering the sound "haaah" . . . Let the rest of your body stay relaxed . . . Observe the sensations of tightening. Now let go and relax . . . Observe the contrast in feeling between the clenched fist and the relaxed hand . . . Observe the difference in the way your right and left hands feel now.

Now tighten your left fist . . . Observe the sensations of tightening. Keep breathing slowly and diaphragmatically; let the rest of your body stay soft and relaxed . . . Now let go. Observe the sensations and feelings of letting go . . . If your attention wanders to other things, gently bring it back to the sensations in your hand and arm.

Now tighten both fists . . . Observe the sensations of tightening . . . Now let go and relax all over . . . Enjoy the sensation . . . Notice the difference between the tension and relaxation.

Now bend your arms at your elbows . . . Tense both biceps (the muscles in the front of your upper arms) . . . Let your hands and fingers stay relaxed . . . Observe the sensations of tightening . . . Keep breathing . . . slowly . . . and deeply . . Let your neck, your jaw, and the rest of your body be soft and relaxed . . . Now relax and let your arms drop to your side or onto your lap . . . Notice the difference in the feelings of tensing and letting go.

Straighten your arms in front of you and hold them parallel to the floor so that you tense your triceps muscles (the muscles in the back of your upper arms) . . . Let your hands stay relaxed; keep breathing slowly and easily . . . Observe the sensations of tightening . . . Now let your arms drop to your sides or into your lap . . . Relax all over . . . Notice that your arms feel comfortable and heavy . . . Feel the relaxation spread up your arms . . . Notice that your arms feel heavier and heavier as you relax more and more.

Now frown hard, letting the rest of your body stay relaxed . . . Now relax and let go . . . Wrinkle your eyebrows up toward your scalp, while letting your tongue, jaw, and neck stay soft and loose . . . Keep breathing slowly and deeply . . . Observe the sensation of tightening . . . Relax and let your brow be smooth . . . Observe the sensations of relaxation.

Now tighten your eyes . . . Tighten the muscles deep in your eyes and tighten the facial muscles around your eyes . . . Let your tongue, your jaw, the back of your neck, and the rest of your body stay relaxed . . . Now relax your eyes and keep them gently closed . . . Observe the sensations of relaxation and how they differ from those of tightening.

Clench your jaw and teeth . . . Notice the tension in your jaw . . . Keep breathing slowly and easily. Now relax and let go . . . Part your lips slightly as you exhale and let the air flow out of your mouth in a soft whispered "haaahhhhhh."

Press your tongue hard against the roof of your mouth . . . Observe the tension . . . Now relax and let go . . . Feel the relaxation in your cheeks, scalp, eyes, face, arms, hands.

Now tighten your neck by pulling your chin toward your chest . . . Keep breathing slowly and easily, let the rest of your body stay soft and relaxed . . . Feel the tension in your neck. Relax and let go . . . Breathe comfortably, and let your jaw stay relaxed.

Raise your shoulders to your ears, letting your neck and the rest of your body stay relaxed . . . Notice the contrast in how your shoulders feel and how the rest of your body feels . . . Relax and let go, letting the relaxation flow into your back, neck, throat, jaw, and face . . . Let it go deeper and deeper . . . Feel the force of gravity pulling on your body.

Now breathe slowly and deeply and hold your breath . . . Notice the tension in your chest and shoulders . . . Now allow your shoulders to let go, even while you still hold your breath; let your eyes, your jaw, and the rest of your body be relaxed . . . Now exhale and observe the feelings . . . Breathe in and out normally, and notice that with each exhalation you feel more and more relaxed . . . Let your chest be loose and soft as you breathe out.

Now take another deep breath . . . Hold your breath but let your neck be relaxed . . . Now exhale and feel yourself let go of the tension . . . Let the relaxation spread to your shoulders, neck, back, and arms.

Now tighten your stomach . . . Make it solid . . . Now relax and notice the well-being that accompanies your relaxation . . . Now suck your stomach in and hold it . . . Relax and let go . . . Let your breathing go slowly and easily, in and out . . . Notice your whole lower abdomen moving out as you inhale . . . Notice how exhaling relaxes your shoulders, chest, and stomach. Let go of all the tension in your body.

Arch your lower back so there is a space between your back and the chair or floor . . . Feel the tension along your spine and back . . . Let your legs and the rest of your body stay relaxed . . . Now relax and let go . . . Relax your lower back, upper back, stomach, chest, shoulders, arms, face, relaxing further and further.

Tighten your buttocks; be sure your abdomen and the rest of your body are relaxed . . . Keep breathing slowly and gently . . . Now relax and let go . . . Feel how different the sensations of relaxation are from those of tension.

Pull your knees together slightly and tighten your thighs . . . Now let the knees separate and allow the legs to relax . . . Now point your toes and feet downward to tighten your calves and the arches of your feet but not so much as to cause cramping . . . Keep breathing . . . Relax and let go . . . Curl your toes toward your knees to create tension along your shins and the tops of your feet . . . Relax and let go.

Now let go more and more of each of the parts of your body: feet relax . . . ankles relax . . . calves . . . shins . . . knees . . . and thighs relax . . . buttocks and hips . . . Feel the heaviness of your lower body . . . and stomach relax . . . waist and lower back relax . . . Let go more and more and breathe easily . . . upper back relax . . . chest relax . . . shoulders and arms relax . . . Let relaxation take over . . . throat relax . . . neck . . . jaws . . . and face relax.

When you are ready, take a deep breath, slowly sit up, and gently open your eyes. Observe how you feel and how you perceive your environment. Do you notice a difference in brightness, clarity, vividness, aliveness, depth of vision?

Each day after you have gone through the script, complete **Log Sheet: Practice 2**. If you experience an incongruous response or an extreme physical or psychological response, refer to the section, "Important Variables to Optimize Training" in Chapter 1. At the end of the week answer **Questions: Practice 2**. Meet with your group and complete **Discussion and Conclusions: Practice 2**.

Name _____ Date _____

Log Sheet   Dynamic Relaxation: Practice 2

After each practice, describe (a) the practice situation (your mood, the place, your physical position, etc.) and (b) your physical and emotional experiences both during and directly following your practice.

Day 1   a. _____

Date _____   _____

_____

_____

             b. _____

_____

_____

_____

Day 2   a. _____

Date _____   _____

_____

             b. _____

_____

_____

_____

Day 3   a. _____

Date _____   _____

_____

             b. _____

_____

_____

_____

Day 4   a. _____
Date _____ _____
              _____

              b. _____
              _____
              _____
              _____

Day 5   a. _____
Date _____ _____
              _____

              b. _____
              _____
              _____
              _____

Day 6   a. _____
Date _____ _____
              _____

              b. _____
              _____
              _____
              _____

Day 7   a. _____
Date _____ _____
              _____

              b. _____
              _____
              _____
              _____

Describe the ritual by which you begin the relaxation practice:

_____
_____
_____

44

Name _____ Date _____

Questions   Dynamic Relaxation: Practice 2

1. What benefits occurred as a result of your practice?

_____

_____

_____

_____

2. Did your experiences with Dynamic Relaxation vary during the sessions? If so, how did these differences relate to the conditions under which you practiced? (Example: It was difficult to maintain attention during practice at the end of the day.)

_____

_____

_____

_____

3. Did you notice that you held your breath and/or tightened muscles other than the intended muscle during your practice? Which ones? How did your ability to selectively tighten muscles change over the week?

_____

_____

_____

_____

4. What problems/challenges, if any, occurred?

_____

_____

_____

5. How did you solve the problems/challenges?

_____

_____

_____

Name_____ Date_____

Discussion and Conclusions   Dynamic Relaxation: Practice 2

1. What benefits did the group members notice as a result of the practices?

_____

_____

_____

_____

_____

2. What rituals that the other participants used might you adapt for your own
   use?

_____

_____

_____

_____

_____

3. What creative solutions to problems emerged from the group?

_____

_____

_____

_____

_____

4. Topics for which instructor consultation would be helpful:

_____

_____

_____

_____

List your group members: _____ _____

_____ _____ _____

_____ _____ _____

BREATHING: THE MIND–BODY BRIDGE: PRACTICE 3[3]

Breath is the bridge which connects life to consciousness, which unites your body to your thoughts.

THICH NHAT HANH

Show me how you breathe, and I'll show you how you live . . .

ANONYMOUS

Consider the following words and expressions: don't breathe a word; don't waste your breath; breathtaking; sigh of relief; breath of fresh air; with bated breath; breathless; long-winded; to breathe life into; the breath of life.

Breathing is an essential process for human life. Breath patterns influence our physiology, our psychological state, and our unconscious. We are, however, most often unaware of our breathing. Breathing is under both conscious and unconscious control, thus serving as a bridge between the two and a way of learning that mind and body are not separate. Breath (*qi, chi, prana*) in many philosophical systems is considered the vital link to energy, awareness, and transcendence. Think of the double meaning of the words *inspire* and *expire*.

Because breathing reflects both your emotional and physical state, quieting your breathing will soothe your emotions and mental processes as well as calm your body. Many performers, including athletes and musicians, use diaphragmatic breathing as an essential part of their training to perform at peak level. Diaphragmatic breathing will affect all areas of your life, some subtle and some very obvious.

The Physiology of Breathing

Breathing is a natural process that occurs without conscious control. Babies and young children breathe effortlessly. Most of the movement associated with their breathing occurs primarily in the lower abdominal area: As they exhale, the abdomen goes in slightly; when they inhale the abdomen expands outward and to the sides. Most adults, however, no longer breathe in this healthy pattern. Instead, they hold their abdomen rigid or slack and use a significant amount of upper body muscular activity to inhale.

The major muscle involved in proper breathing is called the diaphragm. This is a dome-shaped muscle located beneath the ribs and above the abdomen. In order to inhale, the diaphragm descends and flattens. This activity displaces (pushes down on) the liquid contents of the abdomen and thereby creates a larger space in the chest. As this space is created, the pressure in the atmosphere exceeds the pressure in the chest and air flows in to balance these pressures, as shown in Figure 2.1. To exhale, the diaphragm must relax and be raised upward, compressing the air in the chest and allowing the air to go out. Thus, inhalation requires that the abdominal area relax and expand, while exhalation requires the abdominal area to decrease in diameter. The chest and shoulders should stay relaxed throughout the breathing cycle.

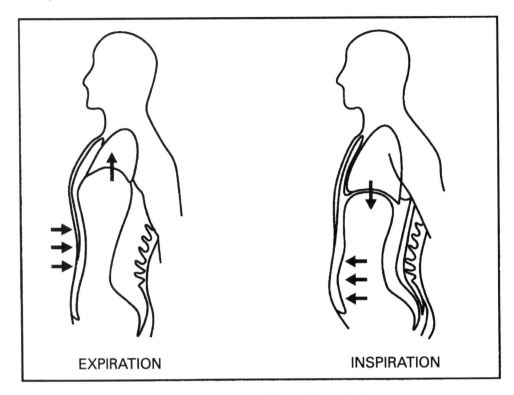

EXPIRATION   INSPIRATION

FIGURE 2.1. Breathing while standing or sitting.

Breathing While Lying Down Versus Sitting Up. The muscular efforts involved in breathing are different when you are lying down than when you are sitting up. When you are lying on your back, gravity acts to push your abdomen in. Therefore, when you inhale your diaphragm descends, which pushes your abdomen outward. You perceive this as effort. Exhaling is effortless because gravity pushes your abdomen down and thereby pushes your diaphragm upward into your chest, as shown in Figure 2.2. When you are sitting or standing, a slight effort is required to pull the abdomen in so that the diaphragm is pushed back up at end of the exhalation. Inhalation in the vertical position is effortless since you just relax the abdominal wall and allow the diaphragm to go down.

Dysfunctional (Unhealthy) Breathing Patterns.

I found that I would really allow myself to get caught up in the feeling of the moment, and it was at these times that I would stop breathing, and feel my body tense up. I was able by the end of the practice to focus in those moments of fear or pain and to breathe them through, instead of keeping them inside myself to fester. I found that this exercise has also helped my self-confidence.

STUDENT

There are two major breath patterns that are associated with a sense of breath-

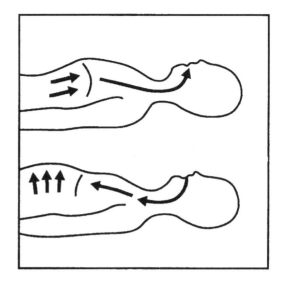

Stomach falls due to gravity for effortless exhalation

Stomach expands with a slight effort during inhalation

FIGURE 2.2. Breathing while lying down.

lessness and/or illness: thoracic breathing and hyperventilation. Both patterns occur with episodic breath holding. These patterns may be very obvious or quite subtle. Even the subtle forms, however, can be deleterious to health.

The first pattern, thoracic breathing, includes shallow breathing punctuated by breath holding or gasping. This unconscious pattern involves the alarm and startle reactions, meaning that the abdomen tightens and the person inhales into the upper chest. The physiological effects of this pattern include increased heart rate, increased blood pressure, gastrointestinal distress symptoms, respiratory symptoms, and neck and shoulder tension. Habitually breathing in this pattern fosters illness. When we are learning something new, the anxiety of the learning

Physiological Changes Associated with Breathing

Thoracic Breathing		Diaphragmatic Breathing
↑	Heart Rate	↓
↑	Blood Pressure	↓
↑	Risk for Heart Attack	↓
↑	Sweat Response	↓
↑	Gastrointestinal Distress	↓
↑	Panic	↓
↑	Hyperventilation Symptoms	↓
↓	Relaxation	↑
↓	Peripheral Temperature	↑

↑ = increases
↓ = decreases

situation often causes dysfunctional breathing. This breathing pattern then becomes associated (conditioned) with the newly learned behavior. One participant observed that each time she wrote in shorthand, she breathed shallowly and remembered how stressful it was to learn shorthand. In your daily logs you will be asked to observe when you gasp or hold your breath.

The second pattern, hyperventilation, is characterized by rapid, shallow breathing punctuated by frequent sighs. When one hyperventilates, too much carbon dioxide is expired, which increases the alkalinity of the blood. Anxiety, phobias, dizziness, and hypertension are all associated with hyperventilation. We commonly think of hyperventilation as an acute and very noticeable state; however, it is often both subtle and chronic.

Symptoms of Chronic Hyperventilation[4]

Respiratory: Asthma, tight chest, dyspnea (breathlessness), excessive sighing or yawning, dry cough, shortness of breath.

Cardiovascular: Palpitations, tachycardia (rapid heart rate), chest pain or angina, Raynaud's disease (blood vessel constriction in the hands and/or feet).

Neurological: Dizziness, faintness, migraines, numbness, intolerance of bright lights or loud noise.

Gastrointestinal: Dysphagia (difficulty in swallowing), dry throat, gas, belching, globus (lump in the throat), abdominal discomfort.

Muscular: Cramps, tremors, twitches, muscle pain.

Psychological: Tension, anxiety, phobias.

General: Fatigue, exhaustion, weakness, lack of concentration and memory, sleep disturbances, nightmares.

Advantages of Diaphragmatic Breathing and Disadvantages of Thoracic Breathing.   All our physiological processes are controlled by the nervous system. One branch of the nervous system, called the sympathetic nervous system (SNS), is strongly affected by how we breathe. When we breathe rapidly, shallowly, and in our chests (thoracically), the sympathetic nervous system becomes activated. This results in increased heart rate and blood pressure, cool hands and feet, sweaty palms, and other symptoms. People who habitually breathe this way may experience a sense of panic and symptoms associated with hyperventilation; they may even increase their risk of heart attacks. People who suffer from panic attacks almost always have this breathing pattern.

Emotions have a profound effect on breathing patterns. When we are startled, we often gasp and/or hold our breath. The startle or alarm reaction then leads to increased sympathetic nervous system arousal and all the physiological changes associated with that arousal.

Slow diaphragmatic breathing, on the other hand, decreases the sympathetic nervous system activity and encourages regeneration. Slow diaphragmatic breathing has been shown to reduce by half the occurrence of a coronary event in people who have already suffered a heart attack (van Dixhoorn et al., 1987). It also results in lowered blood pressure and heart rate, warm hands and feet, a decreased sweat response, and a general sense of relaxation and well-being.

Reminders and Suggestions

- Breathe "low and slow." Let your awareness be deep in your abdomen, below the navel.
- Eliminate the "designer jeans syndrome." If you wear constricting clothing, experiment with loosely fitting styles this week.
- Do not alter the use of your medication without consulting your health care provider.
- If you feel faint as you practice any of the exercises, stop the practice. Allow yourself to gently focus on the very slow exhalation. To help you lengthen an exhalation, try letting the air out with a "Ssssss" sound as if exhaling through a very tiny opening. The sound itself will help to remind you to slow your breathing.
- Do not try too hard at any time. Practice all exercises at a 70% effort rather than 100%. The purpose is to learn at your own pace, not to be perfect.
- Under stress always exhale first before taking the next breath.
- Do not expect instant success. Be patient. The skills to be learned may take many weeks or even months to master. When you first begin breathing diaphragmatically, you may experience a reduction of skill in some areas. For example, when you first begin to breathe diaphragmatically, speaking may feel awkward and impossible. Or when breathing diaphragmatically while performing music, you may initially feel distracted from the playing, and your performance may suffer. This happens because the arm/hand movements involved with playing the instrument were learned with thoracic breathing; you are now relearning the skill in association with the new, healthier breathing pattern. Do not be alarmed; you will find that your new skill level will exceed the previous level in time because diaphragmatic breathing helps you to release dysfunctional muscle tension and lower your stress arousal.
- Be gentle with yourself and remember that it is normal to have emotions surface when you slow your breathing down. In rare cases, you may find that you experience strong emotions when you allow yourself to breathe diaphragmatically. This may be either an uncomfortable or a positive experience.
- If you have difficulty feeling the movement of breath in your abdomen, you might try looking in a mirror while breathing.
- To deepen your awareness, take three slow diaphragmatic breaths before getting out of bed each morning while saying to yourself, "Today is a new day."

Specific Instructions before Beginning Breathing Practice

Before beginning this practice, be sure that you will have uninterrupted quiet time for at least 20 minutes in a comfortable room. This practice begins in a sitting posture and progresses to a lying-down position.

For the sitting position, sit in a comfortable chair, preferably one providing good lower back support. Place both feet on the floor, with knees slightly apart. (If your feet do not touch the floor, you might put a phone book under them, or whatever is handy.) Loosen your belt or waistband, and even undo your zipper part way to allow plenty of breathing room.

For the lying position, choose a comfortable surface such as a bed or a rug. Lie on your back with your feet shoulder-width apart and your arms a few inches away from the body. Be sure you are comfortable; try placing one pillow under your knees for lower back support and one under your head. Then be ready to place a 2 to 5-pound weight on your abdomen. This can be a book or a bag of rice or beans (we recommend a plastic bag of rice or beans because it conforms to the curve of the abdomen and is less likely to slide off).

As you listen to the tape, simply allow the suggestions to be guidelines for you. Listen to your own rhythm. For example, your exhalations may be longer or shorter than suggested by the script. Many people try too hard at first. Remember, your goal is EFFORTLESS breathing and you are using breathing to help you become quiet and peaceful.

Diaphragmatic Breathing Script

Sit comfortably and begin by stroking your abdomen gently to bring your awareness there and to help you let go of tense, tight muscles. Breathe as you stroke, for the next few minutes. You may close your eyes in order to bring awareness to your breathing . . . .

Now place one hand over your lower abdomen and one on your chest and breathe comfortably through your nose . . . Use your hands to help you become aware of your breathing, to help you notice where your body moves as the air flows in and out. What do you feel? . . . As you breathe out, make a soft whispered "Haaaa" sound . . . Allow your shoulders to stay relaxed.

At the end of your next exhalation, slightly pull in your abdominal muscles to help you exhale a little more while whispering "Haaaa." Then let the air flow in passively, no effort needed . . . Slowly and gently inhale through your nose and exhale through your mouth whispering "Haaaa." . . . Notice any tension in your abdomen and let it go.

Breathe at your own rhythm, gently and slowly . . . Feel your abdomen moving with your hand . . . As you breathe out, think of pulling your abdomen in a tiny bit at the end of the exhalation. Just do this for the next few breaths.

As you breathe in, feel your whole abdomen widening and the pelvis opening up . . . Feel the movement in the lower part of your back as you inhale . . . Then let the air out slowly and comfortably while whispering "Haaaa." . . . Continue for a few minutes . . .

Now as you breathe in, imagine a large beach ball in your abdomen that is filling more and more with air as you inhale . . . Then feel it deflating as you exhale . . . Imagine this for a few breaths . . . Notice the internal feelings with the expanding and contracting of the beach ball . . . Continue to breathe and feel the beach ball for a few minutes . . . .

Now while you continue to breathe easily, take a moment to open your eyes and notice how your body feels . . .

Now gently move to your lying-down position and make sure you are comfortable . . . Place the weight on your abdomen, over your navel, and simply observe what it feels like as you breathe in and out . . . Allow your eyes to close . . . Feel your abdomen moving as you inhale and pushing the weight upon . . . As you exhale feel your abdomen becoming flat and the weight pushing the air out . . . Now inhale and push the weight up, and as you exhale allow the weight to push your air out . . . Allow the air to flow evenly and slowly . . . Feel the weight rising and your abdomen expanding during inhalation and the weight sinking and your abdomen flattening during exhalation. Continue this breathing for a few minutes . . . .

Become aware of how slowly you are breathing . . . Then gradually begin to lengthen the exhalation by silently counting to yourself: exhaling . . . 2 . . . 3 . . . 4 . . . Let all the air out and then let the breath flow in easily . . . Let it go slowly and comfortably . . . As you count, let the numbers gradually increase . . . Allow the exhalation to lengthen as your body settles into peacefulness . . . Allow the air to flow in and out your nose for the next few minutes while you count the duration of the exhalation.

Allow your breath to relax your body. Just breathe slowly, fully, easily . . . Give yourself permission to let go . . . Now let go of the counting and for the next few minutes say to yourself, "As I breathe in, I am aware I'm breathing in. As I breathe out, I am aware I'm breathing out."

Finally, imagine yourself lying on a beach and hearing the rhythmic sound of the waves . . . Let your breathing be like the waves, flowing in and out, a timeless natural rhythm, a ceaseless ebb and flow . . . receding and moving out toward the horizon . . . Be one with the wave . . . Let all tension flow away from you. Feel a warm wave of relaxation spreading through your whole body.

Allow yourself to relax a few minutes longer, just keeping your awareness on the flow of your breath as it goes in and out . . . When you are ready, wiggle your fingers and toes, give yourself a gentle stretch, and open your eyes. Note your feelings of calm; allow them to go with you as you breathe effortlessly through the rest of your day.

Each day, after you have gone through the script, complete **Log Sheet: Practice 3**. At the end of the week, answer **Questions: Practice 3**. Meet with your group and complete **Discussion and Conclusions: Practice 3**.

Name _____ Date _____

Log Sheet   Diaphragmatic Breathing: Practice 3

Each day describe (a) your experience and effects of practicing the script (tape):
(b) situations during your daily activities where you gasped or held your breath,
such as while driving or while chopping vegetables; and (c) your experience of
the event or activity when you changed to slow diaphragmatic breathing.

Day 1   a. _____

Date _____   _____

_____

               b. _____

_____

               c. _____

_____

Day 2   a. _____

Date _____   _____

_____

               b. _____

_____

               c. _____

_____

Day 3   a. _____

Date _____   _____

_____

               b. _____

_____

               c. _____

_____

Day 4   a. _____

Date _____   _____

_____

b. _____

_____

c. _____

_____

Day 5   a. _____

Date _____   _____

_____

b. _____

_____

c. _____

_____

Day 6   a. _____

Date _____   _____

_____

b. _____

_____

c. _____

_____

Day 7   a. _____

Date _____   _____

_____

b. _____

_____

c. _____

_____

Name _____ Date _____

Questions   Diaphragmatic Breathing: Practice 3

1. What benefits occurred as a result of your practice?

_____
_____
_____
_____
_____

2. Under what situations did you gasp or hold your breath?

_____
_____
_____
_____
_____

3. In what ways did the shift into diaphragmatic breathing change your experience?

_____
_____
_____
_____
_____

4. What problems/challenges occurred?

_____
_____
_____

5. How did you solve the problems/challenges?

_____
_____
_____

Name_____ Date_____

Discussion and Conclusions   Diaphragmatic Breathing: Practice 3

1. What benefits did the group members notice as a result of the practices?

_____

_____

_____

_____

_____

_____

2. How did the experiences that occurred during and following the breathing practice vary among group members? Was there any association between these differences and age, gender, medical background, previous experience with relaxation techniques, etc.?

_____

_____

_____

_____

_____

3. What were the common themes associated with gasping and breath holding and attempted change by continued slow diaphragmatic breathing?

_____

_____

_____

_____

_____

5. Topics for which instructor consultation would be helpful:

_____

_____

List your group members: _____ _____

_____ _____ _____

_____ _____ _____

DEVELOPING A PERSONAL RELAXATION IMAGE: PRACTICE 4

Physically creating my personal relaxation scene through watercolors was more impactful than relying solely on imagination. It became a powerful and cathartic exercise pulling up chains of strong affective associations complete with smells, sounds, and feelings that had been blocked off from childhood. These memories felt as strong in my system as certain drugs. These memories were then integrated into my practice and directly contributed to the positive results I had.

STUDENT

I enjoyed regressing back into my childhood, playing in the rain, making paper sailboats with my brother . . . Placing my fingers in a bowl of water and stroking a paper sailboat enabled me to participate in the total experience . . . I felt tingling sensations all over my body, much like tiny bundles of energy exploding inside of me. By the end of the week the simple word rain *could induce these sensations inside my whole being.*

STUDENT

Daydreaming! We all know how to do it, and it has much in common with the following beneficial imagery practice. Before beginning the practice, first recall an image of wholeness, as described in the following section (Pavlov Exercise) and then develop your own personalized relaxation image.

Pavlov Exercise

Most of us are probably familiar with the classical conditioning experiment of Ivan Pavlov, the famous Russian physiologist. He found that he was able to teach dogs to salivate when they heard a bell ring, even when no food was provided to them. Pavlov accomplished this by giving the dogs food immediately after ringing the bell for a certain period of time. Eventually, they became conditioned to expect the food with the bell: simply hearing the bell ring would induce salivation.

There is a story about Pavlov[5] that as an old man he became quite ill with heart disease. His doctors had no hope of curing him, so they took his family aside and told them that the end was near. Pavlov himself, however, was not disheartened. He asked the nurse who was caring for him to bring him a bowl of warm water with a bit of mud in it. All day as he lay in bed, he dabbled one hand in the water with a dreamy, faraway look on his face. His family was quite sure that he had taken leave of his wits and would soon die. However, the next morning he announced that he felt fine, ate a large breakfast, and sat out in the sun awhile; by the end of the day, when the doctor came to check on him, there was no trace of the serious heart condition. When asked to explain what he had done, Pavlov said that he had reasoned that if he could recall a time when he was completely carefree and happy, it might have some healing benefit for him. As a young boy he used to spend his summers playing with his friends in a shallow swimming hole in a nearby river. The memory of the warm, slightly muddy water was delightful to him. With his knowledge of the power of conditioned stimuli, Pavlov decided that having a physical reminder of that water would help him evoke that time and those blissful feelings and bring the memories into present time. And that was how he harnessed positive emotions to bring about his healing.

Each of us performs many conditioned behaviors every day. Some of these behaviors can have significant implications for our health and wellness. For example, some components of certain allergic reactions may be conditioned. One woman developed a severe allergic reaction to a very realistic-looking paper rose, although she was not allergic to paper. She did, however, know that she was allergic to roses and reacted to what she believed was a rose (Mackenzie, 1886).

Another example is an experiment that showed that rats can be conditioned to suppress their immune systems. The rats were injected with a powerful immune-suppressing drug while being fed saccharin-flavored water. Their immune function was then measured, and it showed an immediate drop. After the drug and saccharine water were paired a number of times, these rats were given just the saccharin water and a harmless injection of salt water. But their immune cells responded exactly as if they had received the drug! The reverse ability, increasing immune cell functioning, was also shown to be learnable through conditioning (Ader & Cohen, 1975; Ghanta et al., 1985).

Developing Pavlov's Exercise

In this exercise you will be asked to think back to a time when you felt joy, peace, or a sense of integration/wholeness. For some this might be a short moment while for others it could be an extended time period. You will then be asked to become very relaxed as you think of that time and the feelings and sensations associated with feeling well, evoking as many senses as possible. The goal is to pair the experience of relaxation with the feeling of health and well-being. Just as unhealthy behaviors can be conditioned, so too can healthy responses. If possible, have with you an actual object, picture, or smell (such as an old teddy bear, a shell from the beach, a favorite song, a certain perfume—olfactory and gustatory cues can be especially powerful) from that previous time period. This will often facilitate evoking the memory.

Suggestions

During this week's practice, first develop your own personal relaxation/healing image and describe it. Then practice the exercise. Relax and let go. Observe the changes in your sensations.

This time we will reduce the number of steps involved in relaxing by combining muscle groups. You will also begin to use cue words and images to encourage relaxation. If English is not your native language, you may choose to use a word or phrase from your mother tongue that elicits, represents, or is associated with a sense of wholeness. If you're having trouble isolating a muscle, touch it or stroke it with your hands and then tense it and feel the tension in your hands; feel the difference, with your hands, as you let go of the tension. Or you may tighten less, only as much as is needed to feel the tension.

Occasionally practice this and the next few scripts with your eyes open. This will help you to transfer the relaxation skills into normal everyday life. Also, notice your posture this week. How do you hold yourself? Do you habitually slump forward while studying or working? Do you create tension in your neck, shoulders, or spine?

For this week's practice, prepare for relaxation by unplugging the telephone; adjusting the heat to a comfortable temperature; ensuring that you will have uninterrupted quiet time for 20 to 30 minutes; loosening any constricting clothing; removing jewelry, glasses, and so on; and settling into a comfortable chair, bed, or wherever you can easily relax (refer to your Checklist for Relaxation Practice, p. 38.

When you visualize your Personal Relaxation Image, picture it in your mind's eye and fill in all the details. See the colors, shapes, and textures that you delight to see; feel the texture of the ground under your feet and the temperature of the air on your skin. Make it vivid for yourself, so vivid that you can even hear the sounds of the place—or even just stillness. Are there any fragrances or aromas that you associate with this beautiful place? Can you imagine them? And now see yourself—and feel yourself—strolling easily and slowly through this lovely place, taking in the sights and scents and sounds and letting the peacefulness soak into your being. Imagine yourself settling down in the most comfortable, secure spot.

Using significant elements (images, odors, tastes, sounds) from your imagery of wholeness worksheet, if possible, have with you a sensory reminder or cue to help evoke the memory and the experience of wholeness. For your Personal Relaxation Image, create a scene that you find especially relaxing and one that engenders a sense of wholeness and trust. Stay in your image: see it, smell it, taste it, touch it, be it. This may be similar to or different from your imagery of wholeness. Stay focused on an image that is particularly relaxing and peaceful. Go with the image and allow the relaxation to deepen.

First complete the **Worksheet: Imagery of Wholeness: Practice 4.** Then create your own personal relaxation scene. Describe it on **Worksheet: Personal Relaxation Image: Practice 4.** When you are making your tape for the personal relaxation script, substitute your own Personal Relaxation Image (from the worksheet on p. 64) for the indented text sample image in the script.

Optional: Get a massage. Compare your level of relaxation afterward to the result of this practice. What muscles are chronically tight? Do some gentle stretches or "shake out" your limbs, just before doing your relaxation practice.

Draw or paint the relaxing image or actually go to your "relaxing place" (if possible) and do your practice. Practice outdoors in the most relaxing place you can find. Nature is a healer.

Return to your Personal Relaxation Image for just a few seconds during the day to evoke a sense of peace.

Worksheet   Imagery of Wholeness: Practice 4

1. Identify a time in your past when you felt joy, peace, or a sense of integration/wholeness.

   _____

   _____

   _____

   _____

2. Describe the specific cues or stimuli that could be used to evoke the wholeness image.

   _____

   _____

   _____

   _____

   _____

   _____

3. Describe in detail the image that you associate with wholeness.

   _____

   _____

   _____

   _____

   _____

   _____

   _____

   _____

   _____

   _____

   _____

   _____

Name_____ Date_____

Worksheet   Personal Relaxation Image: Practice 4

Write out the script for your personal relaxation image.

_____

_____

_____

_____

_____

_____

_____

_____

_____

_____

_____

_____

_____

_____

_____

_____

_____

_____

_____

_____

_____

_____

_____

_____

_____

_____

A Personal Relaxation Image Script

Begin by getting into a comfortable position for relaxation. Now tense both arms by making fists, and extend both your arms while continuing to breathe . . . Study the tension and let the rest of your body stay relaxed . . . Now relax and let your arms flop down like a rag doll's . . . Become aware of any sensations in your arms and hands.

Now hunch up your shoulders toward your ears and tighten your neck, while keeping your abdomen and jaw loose . . . Continue to breathe easily . . . and allow your shoulders to drop. Feel the relaxation flowing from your shoulders down your arms, breathing slowly and comfortably.

Squeeze your eyes shut tight, press your lips and teeth together, and wrinkle up your nose; feel the tightness in your whole face . . . Notice if tension creeps back into your upper body; if it does, let it go . . . Now relax your face, let it soften, and feel the sensations of letting go . . . Feel your breath coming in and out.

Now press your shoulders backward and tighten up your chest and stomach at the same time . . . Let your jaw and thighs be relaxed . . . Let go; let your body sink comfortably into the surface on which you are resting . . . Let yourself relax more with every breath.

Tighten your buttocks, thighs, calves, and feet by pressing your heels down into the floor while curling your toes and squeezing your knees together . . . Feel the tension while continuing to breathe . . . Relax and let go . . . Allow relaxation to flow through your legs . . . Enjoy the feelings of letting go and notice your sensations.

Feel the deepening relaxation, the calmness and the serenity . . . Observe the ease with which your breath is flowing . . . Feel the flowing of the relaxation . . . Let the feeling deepen as you relax more . . . Notice the developing sense of inner confidence and the calm indifference to external events . . . Now deepen the relaxation even further by mentally repeating any word or phrase you associate with feelings of calm, wholeness, and relaxation . . . For example, "I am relaxed" . . . "I am loved" . . . or just the word "secure" . . . Say it to yourself slowly as you exhale.

Let your entire body become more and more relaxed. Let the feelings of relaxation, calmness, and serenity deepen for a few minutes . . . Think and feel the words *relax, calm, serene,* or your own special phrase as you exhale . . . Just attend to the relaxation in your body . . . Make sure that no tension has crept back into your head and scalp . . . Relax your forehead, eyes, face, lips, tongue, and jaw. Let your whole body be relaxed . . . Let relaxation spread through your neck, shoulders, and arms . . . down your sides . . . and through your chest, stomach, lower back, knees, calves, ankles, and feet . . . Let your entire body relax more and more deeply, as you repeat your special words with each exhalation.

Now allow an image to form in your mind of a beautiful place in nature where you can feel completely comfortable, secure, warm, joyous, and relaxed . . . It might be a beach on a sunny day or a quiet, peaceful meadow surrounded by woods or any place at all—real or imaginary.

Insert your Personal Relaxation Image here or continue with the following sample image script.

> You are walking through a mountain meadow after having emerged from a cool, dark forest. Here and there the green grass is dotted with brightly colored wildflowers in hues of pink, yellow, red, and purple. Touch the delicate petals of a flower and inhale its fresh, sweet fragrance . . . Remove your shoes and socks and let your feet feel the cool, moist softness of the thick grass. Feel the sun overhead warming your shoulders and arms while a gentle breeze tousles your hair and soothes your forehead . . . In the distance hear an occasional clear note of a bird's song breaking the silence. A butterfly lazily dips and floats among the flowers and grasses. Smell the grass and a faint scent of pine needles. . .
>
> As you walk along, enjoying the springy grasses underfoot, become aware of the sound of a brook, which grows louder as you approach . . . For a while watch and listen as the water bubbles swiftly over the mossy stones . . . The sun glistens brightly on the moving water. Leaning over, let your fingers dangle for a moment in the clear, cool stream . . . And now relax and settle back comfortably here, for as long as you like . . .

After visualizing this scene or your Personal Relaxation Image, or the sample scene, continue with the script.

Let yourself just stay in this special place all your own, and know that you can return to this peaceful sanctuary any time you choose to do so . . . When you are ready, take a deep breath, gently stretch your body, and open your eyes.

Each day after you have gone through the script, complete **Log Sheet: Practice 4**. At the end of the week, answer **Questions: Practice 4**. Meet with your group and complete **Discussion and Conclusions: Practice 4**.

Name _____ Date _____

Log Sheet   Personal Relaxation Image: Practice 4

For each daily practice session (a) describe the "realness of your imagery" and (b) make notes of your mood and physical state before, during, and after the relaxation.

Day 1   a. _____
Date _____   _____
             _____
             b. _____
             _____
             _____
             _____

Day 2   a. _____
Date _____   _____
             _____
             b. _____
             _____
             _____
             _____

Day 3   a. _____
Date _____   _____
             _____
             b. _____
             _____
             _____
             _____

Day 4   a. _____
Date _____   _____
             _____

            b. _____

_____

_____

_____

Day 5   a. _____

Date _____   _____

_____

            b. _____

_____

_____

_____

Day 6   a. _____

Date _____   _____

_____

            b. _____

_____

_____

_____

Day 7   a. _____

Date _____   _____

_____

            b. _____

_____

_____

_____

Additional comments/questions:

_____

_____

_____

_____

Name _____ Date _____

Questions   Personal Relaxation Image: Practice 4

1. What benefits occurred as a result of your practice?

_____

_____

_____

_____

2. How did the cue words affect your relaxation experience?

_____

_____

_____

_____

3. How did the images affect your relaxation?

_____

_____

_____

_____

4. In which ways was this week's experience different from that of the previous week?

_____

_____

_____

_____

5. What problems/challenges occurred and how did you solve them?

_____

_____

_____

_____

_____

Name _____ Date _____

Discussion and Conclusions   Personal Relaxation Image:
Practice 4

1. What benefits did the group members notice as a result of the practice?

_____

_____

_____

_____

_____

_____

2. Were there common words or images that encouraged or inhibited relaxation?

_____

_____

_____

_____

_____

3. Among group members how were the experiences of this week's practice related to (a) ease of the practice (b) past and/or present health and illness patterns, (c) previous exposure to relaxation or meditation techniques?

_____

_____

_____

_____

_____

4. Topics for which instructor consultation would be helpful:

_____

_____

List your group members: _____ _____

_____ _____ _____

_____ _____ _____

REDUCING THE TENSION AND INCREASING THE AWARENESS: PRACTICE 5

After a number of times of practicing, my body would just let me know it was time to do the exercise. . . . My body just craved the feeling of peacefulness . . . Instead of waiting till I get a headache, now my body lets me know the slightest presence of tension.
PARTICIPANT

Most eye tension comes from judging what I see. I strain to avoid seeing what is there or to see what is not there. Acceptance implies gentler vision. Gentle eyes perceive a gentle world. Tension in my jaw and throat results from judgments also. It occurs when I don't say what I feel or when I say something I don't really feel.
STUDENT

This week the purpose of your practice is to learn to become aware of lesser amounts of tension and then to relax and let them go. Meanwhile, continue to use your cue words to encourage relaxation. As you say your cue words, you may want to visualize your body becoming limp and totally relaxed. Begin this week's practice by tightening each muscle group so that you feel about half the amount of tension that you are capable of exerting. Then let go just as completely as in the last three practices, observing the changes in sensation.

With practice you can become aware of subtle sensations of tension that previously occurred beneath the level of your awareness. By practicing awareness of very subtle tension, you increase your ability to sense when your body is beginning to tighten as you go through your daily activities. As your awareness improves through the week's practice, tighten the muscles just to the point where you can barely feel their tension. This enhanced awareness may help you during the day to prevent the habitual bracing that has been embedded in and conditioned by your daily activity. For example, you might notice such dysponetic activity as a slight tensing of the shoulders and jaw when you play tennis. After reducing the dysponesis, you move more fluidly and improve your performance and endurance.

At the same time, the enhanced awareness of slight tensions during the day can help identify the stressors to which you are reacting. These stressors might consist of external situations and/or thoughts, reactions, and feelings (such as "Oh no! I blew that serve!" or "What a stupid mistake!"). After having identified the stressors, you may choose to relax your tight muscles before discomfort occurs.

Included in this practice session are some specific exercises for the eyes, jaw, and throat, since these are areas in which we often unknowingly hold tension. We often strain our eyes, especially when working for hours at a computer terminal. By doing special gentle exercises for eyes and throat, we bring awareness and greater relaxation to these areas. As you master the skill and grow, be sure to adapt the script to your new state. While practicing, remember:

1. If you are not sure how much to tighten your muscles, tighten them just enough to feel something in the muscles and a sense of letting go when you release them. If you find it difficult to let go of slightly tightened muscles, tighten them more. Give yourself time to increase your skills. You may find

it helpful to go back for a few sessions to Practice 2. Remember: Do not make efforts to reduce efforts.

2. If you experience pain or headaches as a result of the eye or jaw movements, do them with less effort. Most likely, you are straining excessively. Perform the movements very gently and stop if any sense of strain is present. (It is possible that you have chronic tension of the eye or jaw muscles.) Increase the length of time for resting after each movement. While resting, imagine a cool blue light or liquid streaming through the tense areas (such as your eyes or jaw) and soothing them.

Remember to listen to your body to learn when to relax, when to let off steam through exercise, and when to take assertive action. Also talk to your body when you notice muscles tightening. Ask gently, "What am I afraid of? What am I defending against? Can I let go?"

Reducing the Tension and Increasing the Awareness Script

Begin with your relaxation preparations and ritual.

Make sure you are comfortable. Now tighten both fists slightly and continue to breathe easily . . . Let go and relax your arms and fists . . . Notice the difference between tension and relaxation. Remember to tighten only the intended muscles while the rest of your body stays quiet and relaxed . . . Continue to breathe smoothly and effortlessly . . . Each time you let go, let yourself relax further and further.

Tighten your forehead by raising your eyebrows part way . . . Let go and relax . . . Feel your forehead smoothing out . . . Gently squeeze and slightly tighten your eye muscles; feel the sensations . . . Relax your eyes, let them soften . . . Be aware of your easy breathing . . . Tighten your tongue, jaw, and lips, again moderately; feel the tension . . . Let it go completely; feel the loosening and softening taking place . . . Tighten your throat and neck; hold the tension . . . Let go and relax.

While continuing to breathe, raise both arms a few inches, holding them out straight . . . Do this with the least amount of effort. Observe the tension . . . Let it go completely . . . Notice whether any other muscles wanted to tighten up, too . . . Breathe easily.

Raise your shoulders part of the way toward your ears. Observe how your shoulders feel different from the rest of your body . . . Let go and relax . . . Feel the relaxation spreading through your body.

Tighten your stomach muscles a bit and keep breathing slowly and deeply . . . Let go and relax . . . Notice how your abdomen expands as you breathe in . . . Be aware of any slight tensions in your chest and abdomen during your breathing cycle.

Now gently tighten your buttocks partway, while keeping your abdomen relaxed. Breathing deeply and comfortably . . . Now relax and let go . . . Tighten your feet, calves, and thighs halfway . . . Observe the tension level . . . Let go and relax.

Close your eyes and take a few moments to mentally scan over your entire body, just looking for any areas of lingering tension, tightness, or discomfort . . . While breathing slowly and consciously, tighten up any such part of your body once again; hold it and then let it go completely . . . Imagine your breathing is going into those muscles and even helping them relax more.

Bring your awareness back to your eyes now; without straining your eyes and keeping your lids closed, gently look upward . . . Let your jaw and tongue stay loose and relaxed; continue to breathe slowly and easily . . . Relax and let go . . . Now look gently to the left with your eyes closed; hold while you focus your awareness on your breathing . . . Let go . . . Look right with your eyes closed and continue to look right . . . Relax and let go . . . Look downward with your eyelids closed; let your neck, jaw, and tongue stay loose . . . Relax and let go.

Allow your eyes to soften and relax more and more . . . Imagine sensations of coolness in the muscles around your eyes . . . Breathe comfortably and deeply.

While staying totally relaxed, visualize the tip of a pen moving across paper and writing your name very slowly; observe the sensations around and in your eyes . . . Breathe easily; relax and let go; let the image fade from your mind, so that your eyes relax completely . . . Note the sensations around the eyes and gently encourage them to let go, to soften.

Recall an image from your personal relaxation scene and gently observe it in detail . . . Let yourself be surrounded by the experience . . . Let go of the image.

Now direct your attention to the area of your jaw and notice the level of tension present. Close your jaw firmly and observe the tension . . . Let go and relax . . . Open your jaw slowly, gradually, while continuing to breathe, and again notice the level of tension . . . Relax and let go.

Smile and observe the tension; exactly where do you notice tightening? Continue to breathe slowly and comfortably while smiling. Relax and let go . . . Push your tongue against the roof of your mouth; let your eyes and the rest of your face stay relaxed . . . Relax and let go . . . Be aware of your slow, easy breathing.

Now say your name aloud and observe the tightening in your neck and throat . . . Notice the quality of your voice; be aware of your breathing. Relax and let go . . . Say your name in a whisper now; observe which muscles tighten . . . Relax and let go . . . Observe how your throat feels different between the relaxed and tensed state. Let your throat go more and more limp and soft . . . Notice a gentle soothing softness as you relax.

Now just imagine that you are saying your name . . . Observe any tension in your throat as you breathe easily and gently . . . And once again, relax completely.

Repeat your cue word or phrase to yourself and be aware of any throat tension that you might experience as you hear the words in your mind . . . Allow the feelings of calm and relaxation to deepen for a few moments as you repeat the words with each exhalation.

After a few minutes take a deep, energizing breath and stretch your body . . . Gently open your eyes . . . Do you notice a difference in how you see? Is there a difference in brightness, clarity, vividness, and depth in your vision? Speak a few words and observe any differences in the ease, resonance, depth, or softness of your voice.

Optional: Be aware of your facial expressions many times throughout the day. What tensions are present in your face when thinking, reading, talking?

Each day after you have gone through the script, complete **Log Sheet: Practice 5.** At the end of the week answer **Questions: Practice 5.** Meet with your group and complete **Discussion and Conclusions: Practice 5.**

Name _____ Date _____

Log Sheet Reducing the Tension and Increasing the Awareness:
Practice 5

For each daily practice session (a) describe the effect of the practice and (b) the
sense of relaxation of your eyes and throat.

Day 1   a. _____
Date _____   _____
                _____
                _____
             b. _____
                _____
                _____
                _____

Day 2   a. _____
Date _____   _____
                _____
                _____
             b. _____
                _____
                _____
                _____

Day 3   a. _____
Date _____   _____
                _____
                _____
             b. _____
                _____
                _____
                _____

Day 4   a. _____

Date _____   _____

_____

_____

               b. _____

_____

_____

_____

Day 5   a. _____

Date _____   _____

_____

_____

               b. _____

_____

_____

_____

Day 6   a. _____

Date _____   _____

_____

_____

               b. _____

_____

_____

_____

Day 7   a. _____

Date _____   _____

_____

_____

               b. _____

_____

_____

_____

Name _____ Date _____

Questions   Reducing the Tension and Increasing the Awareness:
Practice 5

1. What benefits occurred as a result of your practice?

_____
_____
_____
_____

2. How did your awareness of minimal tension change?

_____
_____
_____
_____

3. What was the effect on your eyes/vision and throat/voice?

_____
_____
_____
_____

4. In which ways were this week's experiences different from those of previous
   weeks?

_____
_____
_____
_____

5. What problems/challenges occurred and how did you solve them?

_____
_____
_____

Name _____ Date _____

Discussion and Conclusions Reducing the Tension and
Increasing the Awareness: Practice 5

1. What benefits did the group members notice as a result of the practice?

_____

_____

_____

_____

_____

_____

2. In which ways did the awareness of minimal tension change?

_____

_____

_____

_____

_____

_____

3. What effects did group members' experience have on eyes/vision and
throat/voice?

_____

_____

_____

_____

4. Topics for which instructor consultation would be helpful:

_____

_____

_____

List your group members: _____ _____

_____ _____ _____

_____ _____ _____

QUICK AND WARM: PRACTICE 6[6]

The secret of health for both mind and body is not to mourn for the past, not to worry about the future, or not to anticipate troubles, but to live the present moment wisely and earnestly.

THE BUDDHA

Learning to relax is not just a withdrawal from the world for 20 minutes. It is introducing relaxation into our daily activities. We get locked into a busy, extremely demanding schedule, and we fear that if we take 20 minutes out we'll get behind. We imagine that if we start slowing down in general, we'll become unproductive, get bored, be judged as unintelligent or, worse, we'll start to see more of who we are and even begin to feel some of the emotional pain that we distract from by staying so busy.

It takes time and personal experience to learn that there is more than one possible way to "be" in the world; that by taking our time we allow more creativity, more quality, in our work and feel more whole and happy and less driven to strive for the outward signs of "success"; and that who we really are is very different from what we thought, and worth getting to know.

While in this transition phase, some quick relaxation methods can be very useful. Charles Stroebel (1982) developed a brief relaxation practice that he called the "quieting reflex," or QR for short. He originally developed it as a result of his own problem with tension headaches. As a busy doctor, he found it hard to take the time out each day for 20 minutes of meditation, progressive relaxation, autogenic training, or other methods that indeed relieved the headaches. He reasoned that since the alarm reaction, or fight-or-flight response, can take place in a few seconds, we should be able to create the relaxation response in an equally brief time. In 6 seconds we can prevent the fight-or-flight response from being activated (except when it is a life-threatening situation, of course) and thus prevent the negative effects of stress. The more frequently it is practiced, the more automatic QR becomes, until it is activated reflexively at a subconscious level whenever we encounter a stressor.

QR can be done in the midst of a stressful situation, with your eyes open, and no one even needs to know you are doing it! With QR you can respond to the situation appropriately without going into an out-of-control stress response. QR can be like a moment of mindfulness, a moment of bringing in space for seeing things differently and for nurturing ourselves when anxious.

QR can be used for preventing anxiety or annoyance, as in preparing for an exam or a confrontation with a problem person. It can help you deal with minor stressors such as stoplights, a ringing telephone, having to wait in line, driving in moderate traffic. Decide to do a QR each time you encounter one of these daily hassles. (One participant initially had trouble relaxing at the sound of a ringing phone; she then decided to laugh at the sound and found that this allowed her to relax and lighten up.)

QR can also be used for habit control: To interrupt the craving, do a QR before lighting a cigarette, taking a drink, or reaching for a snack.

If you are angry, you may quietly clench one fist before doing your QR and really feel the anger before letting it go. When you have strong feelings, acknowledge them and ventilate them safely; don't just QR them away. Once calm, you may be in a better frame of mind to speak assertively (without blowing up). Assertive action is often the key to resolving issues that generate anger.

By now you are becoming aware of your body's responses to stressors, responses such as shallow breathing and tightening of various muscle groups. Scanning your body helps build awareness, which will be very useful in learning QR. Notice how others respond to stress, especially in their body language. Use those responses as cues for a body scan for yourself and for a QR. You may indirectly affect the other person as well, since relaxation can be contagious! After you notice a cue for a QR, say to yourself, "Find something beautiful." Look for the beauty even in a city traffic jam: buildings, colors, sunlight. See your muscle tension as a "point of control" instead of a spiral out of control; take charge—with relaxation.

Here are the steps involved in QR:

1. Become aware of a *cue* (a worry, a feeling of annoyance or anxiety, or muscle tension). Ask yourself, "Is it life threatening?" If not, go on to the next step.
2. Smile inwardly with your mouth and eyes. Let your eyes move to the left and right. Just moving your eyes side to side can remind you that there is more than one way of seeing any situation, no matter how terrible it seems at the moment. Consider that it might even seem amusing to you 5 years from now. Say to yourself, "Alert mind, calm body." Or substitute some other coping phrase, such as "I can relax" or "I can choose peace instead of this." Or just repeat the cue words or phrases that you have been practicing.
3. Inhale a slow, deep abdominal breath. Exhale and let your jaw, tongue, and shoulders go loose. Feel a wave of heaviness flowing through your body, all the way down to your toes.
4. Take another easy breath. Exhale and feel a wave of warmth flowing through your entire body, streaming through your arms and legs as though they were hollow tubes; feel the warm air flowing out your fingers and toes.

That's all there is to it! As Thich Nhat Hanh (1987), a well-known Vietnamese Buddhist meditation teacher, said in his book *Being Peace*: "Breathing in, I calm my body. Breathing out, I smile." During your relaxation practice, incorporate this suggestion with a gentle half smile. Try it now, using a remembered stress cue from your day.

Optional: Smile five times today at people you don't usually smile at: service people, checkout clerks, tolltakers, classmates, complete strangers. What was their response? What was the effect on you?

Deepening Your QR Practice with Hand Warming

In order to receive maximum benefit from your QR practice, it is helpful to have some familiarity and experience with warming your hands. The old phrase "Cold hands, warm heart" might more accurately be changed to "Cold hands, uptight." Peripheral hand temperature is one indication of the level of autonomic arousal. When the sympathetic nervous system is activated, as in the fight-or-flight response, the smooth muscle lining of the peripheral arterioles constricts, causing a decrease in blood flow and thus a drop in hand and foot temperature. Conversely, when the sympathetic nervous system is quiet, these smooth muscles relax, blood flow increases, and hand and foot temperature rises. This is why you may have already noticed your hands warming or tingling when you did slow diaphragmatic breathing or other relaxation exercises in this workbook. In deep relaxation the sympathetic nervous system arousal level drops, leading to peripheral vasodilation and warm hands.

Besides being useful for generalized relaxation, the practice of warming one's hands has been demonstrated to alleviate several other clinical conditions, such as migraine headache, hypertension, Raynaud's disease, and irritable bowel syndrome. Biofeedback training often utilizes a temperature-sensitive indicator for learning the skill of hand warming in order to help people reduce their arousal and relieve these conditions.

Some people react more in certain organ systems than others under stress. For example, some respond with intense skeletal muscle contractions while others respond with smooth muscle contractions. Smooth muscle is found around the arteries (including the coronary arteries), arterioles, and the digestive tract. Thus, people who are "smooth muscle responders" may, for example, develop gastric discomfort, as smooth muscles in the digestive tract constrict; icy cold hands, as their peripheral blood vessels constrict; and chest pain, as the coronary arteries constrict. Migraine headaches are usually preceded by a vasoconstrictive phase—caused by many factors, including stress—in which not only the peripheral blood vessels but also those in the brain constrict; a "rebound vasodilation" then occurs in the head, with throbbing and pain, sometimes accompanied by nausea and vomiting.

For all of these conditions, therefore, an important component of self-regulation is first to become aware of when the smooth muscles constrict (often associated with cooler hands) and, second, to learn to warm your hands. Many researchers, beginning with the pioneering work of Elmer and Alyce Green of the Menninger Foundation, have demonstrated the efficacy of temperature feedback training for hand warming for the treatment of migraine headache.[7] Temperature training was shown useful for regulating high blood pressure by Fahrion, Norris, Green, Green, and Snarr (1986) and by Wittrock, Blanchard, and McCoy (1988); for Raynaud's disease (poor circulation in the hands and feet) by Freedman (1987); and for increasing the healing rate of wounds by Palmer, Tibbetts, and Peper (1991).

Learning that one can warm one's hands—direct one's own blood flow at will—can be an empowering experience. One 13-year-old girl reported that she warmed her hands in the following manner: "I thought to myself that I was in control of everything. Fingers get warm . . . fingers, I feel them warming . . . warm toast, lobsters, ovens, summer . . . I would look at the meter. I would be proud of myself because I had succeeded." Having successfully used this skill to overcome her migraine headaches, she spontaneously generalized the learning process to other body systems. She reported that she told her teeth to move faster so that her orthodontic headgear could come off sooner; the result was that she only had to wear it for 4 months instead of 2 years (Peper & Grossman, 1979). This sense of control can be used to enhance the power of imagery and practice in self-healing. For example, Norris and Porter (1987) report in the book *I Choose Life* the remarkable remission of an inoperable brain tumor in a young boy. He had learned to warm his hands and thus came to experience that he could influence his tumor. Each day he then visualized his immune system's attack upon the tumor until he was healed.

Of course, if you are very warm as you begin a relaxation practice (hand temperature of 94 to 96 degrees Fahrenheit), your hand temperature may drop by a degree or so when you relax in a cooler place or it may simply not change. The maximum finger temperature is generally considered to be 96–97 degrees. The temperature card enclosed with this workbook[8] is not as accurate as the more sensitive temperature biofeedback devices; this is not important, however, as the main thing you need to be aware of is the *relative* changes in temperature.

Increasing Awareness of Blood Flow to Fingers. To begin, the following quick exercises can help you gain an awareness of the sensations of blood flow to your fingers.

To observe the blood flow: While seated, place both hands on your lap. Let them rest there for a few minutes. Observe the color of the two hands. Most likely they are the same color. Now raise your right hand straight up, pointing toward the ceiling. For the next minute hold your right arm up while your left is hanging down at your side. Feel the draining sensation in your right hand and the filling sensation in the left. Then bring both hands to your lap and compare the internal feelings and external color. Note how much lighter your right hand looks. Feel the sensations of blood flowing back into your hand as the color returns.

To push the blood: Stretch your arms up overhead for a moment, then swing them in circles vigorously. Finally let your hands hang down by your sides. Can you feel pulsations or tingling? What color do your hands become?

Attitudes and Strategies to Facilitate Hand Warming. The best attitudinal approach to learning the skill of warming your hands is one of passive attention. The more you try to warm your hands or strive for this goal, the more you will arouse your "efforting mode," which means your sympathetic nervous system becomes activated. It's a lot like trying to produce a urine specimen for the nurse; forcing just doesn't work! Nonjudgmental, passive, open awareness is what lowers your nervous activation. Say to yourself, "If my hands warm up, that's nice, and if they don't, that's okay, too."

When learning the skills of warming your hands, and for relaxation in general, always be sure your body is comfortably warm. Be sure the room is comfortably warm. Many people create unnecessary muscle tension just by not having warm enough clothes as they go about their daily activities. If you are chilly or the room in which you are attempting to relax is cold, warming will be more difficult. Your goal is not to overcome a cold room but to practice deep relaxation. Take a relaxed position, sitting in a comfortable chair or lying down, as for your relaxation practices, with belt loose, glasses off, and so on.

Usually, peripheral temperature will increase through the passive attention. The more you practice, the easier it will become. Simple cue words such as *relax* or *warm* are often helpful while warming your hands. If you find it difficult to allow your hands to warm, check for the following problems and attempt the recommended solutions:

SOME PROBLEMS AND SOLUTIONS

1. *Striving and/or self-judgment.* Acknowledge that it takes time to learn. If possible, think of a peaceful, warm image. Are you trying to "control" your breath? Allow yourself to release it.
2. *Vigilance.* Be sure you are in a safe environment, where you do not need to check your surroundings and will not be disturbed.
3. *Self-consciousness.* Know you have the right to do whatever you want for yourself as long as it does not hurt other people. Explain to the others what you are doing.
4. *Intellectualizing.* Shift your feeling and sensations to your hands and feet. Give or receive a gentle hand massage and just feel the loving sensations.
5. *Excessive heat loss.* Put a scarf and hat on. Much of body heat is lost through the neck and head.
6. *Lack of hand sensations.* Massage your hand or place one of your hands in warm water to experience what the sensation of warmth is. Imagine the other hand warming the same way even though it is not in the water. Or gently tap fingertips together or on a tabletop 50 times. What do you feel? Or rub your hands briskly to generate heat. Exhale gently into cupped palms to experience warmth on exhalation.
7. *Hands cool or no change.* Attempt bidirectional control of hand temperature, and begin by perfecting your skill of hand cooling. Notice what thoughts, images, or feelings help you to cool, such as thinking about an upcoming exam or remembering an unpleasant task or obligation. Then ask yourself, "What is the opposite of these thoughts, images, feelings?" This may give you a clue to the thoughts, images, or feelings that may facilitate warming.
8. *Drafty or uncomfortable location.* Get in a nondrafty location and be sure the chair is comfortable. You might want to turn the heat on in the room to facilitate the peripheral vasodilation. The optimal room temperature for learning is 72 degrees Fahrenheit or higher.
9. *Diurnal rhythms (the body clock).* Practice at different times of day. Later in the afternoon or in the evening, when you have let go of your daily tasks, often works best. Lack of sleep or exhaustion can inhibit the ability to relax and warm.
10. *Metabolic/dietary factors.* Do not consume caffeine (in coffee, colas, chocolate, and black tea). Caffeine induces vasoconstriction. If you are on medications, check whether they are sympathomimetic (capable of increasing autonomic arousal and thus inducing vasoconstriction). In addition, certain foods and liquids may affect peripheral warming; for example,

alcohol often induces hand warming while allergy-causing foods such as milk may induce hand cooling. You may also find it will be easier to warm your hands on a day when you have exercised than on a sedentary day since circulation and metabolic rate are enhanced for hours after exercise. Also, if you have not eaten for a long period of time, warming may be more difficult.

General Instructions for Hand-Warming Exercise. The following scripts emphasize deep relaxation, maintenance of easy diaphragmatic breathing, and hand warming during the tension and relaxation phases of the exercise. This practice implies awareness of your first sensations of stress. *Be sure that during the week you identify the first cues associated with stress.* Then use that awareness to evoke the relaxation. In additon to practicing these scripts, practice QR at least 10 times a day to imprint the habit so that it starts to become automatic. Practice the following exercise for the first day:

For your first experience with temperature observation, take the temperature card enclosed in this book between the thumb and forefinger of your nondominant hand. The nondominant hand and arm sometimes hold less muscle tension, making it easier to observe relaxation and warming in this hand. You will need to wait about a minute in order for the temperature card to equilibriate from the cooler room temperature to the temperature of your fingers. Meanwhile, familiarize yourself with how to read the temperature. After one minute, while still holding the device, record your pre-baseline temperature on your log sheet. Then do the following exercise, which was developed by Norman Cousins (1989).

Suggestion: Usually this exercise will work better if you either tape record the script first and then listen to it or have someone else read it to you.

Script for Hand-Warming Exercise

Day 1

Sit and begin with deep, slow breathing . . . Continue for three or four minutes.

Then think back on your life . . . Think of the nicest thing that happened to you—something that made you feel very good at the time. (Usually, it takes no more than a half-minute for the memory to be summoned.)

Now make this memory as real as possible, so real you can almost taste it. Imagine that you are reliving that experience. Go slowly; breathe deeply . . . Try to feel the way you did during that experience . . . Let everything about that experience give you the same pleasure now that it did then . . . Breathe slowly and deeply. You are feeling very good . . . If the memory makes you laugh or sing out with joy, just do it.

Continue to explore. Imagine that you are able to mobilize your consciousness so that it is like the tip of a blackboard pointer as you move from place to place inside your head. Now let that mobilized consciousness come to rest toward the front of your face, just behind your nose. Concentrate on the tip of your nose . . . Now, imagine the sensation of touching the tip of your nose with your mind. Good. Now, elevate that mobilized consciousness until it comes to rest just behind your eyes. Bear down at the point . . . In a little while you will experience a pulsing sensation behind your eyes.

Now elevate that mobilized consciousness even higher until it comes to rest just under the scalp in the middle of your head. Concentrate at that point. Concentrate hard. In a little while you will experience a slight tingling sensation. (This step generally takes longer than the previous one. When the scalp sensation is experienced, continue.)

Now bring your attention to your hands and allow blood to move into them. You can allow this. Just visualize your heart pumping your blood up to your shoulders, now across the shoulders, and now down your arms, past the elbows, down the forearms, past the wrists, and into your hands . . . Let this flow of warmth into your arms and hands continue.[9]

Record your temperature again. Note what happened and your experience on your daily log.

Days 2 to 7[10]

Begin by taking a comfortable posture. Either tape the thermometer to your index finger or gently hold your temperature device between the thumb and forefinger of your nondominant hand. Observe your temperature after one minute and record your "PRE" temperature on the log sheet. (If it is taped in place, let it stay on for the whole exercise. If you are holding the temperature device, put it down at this time. You will pick it up again at the end of the exercise.)

Allow your eyes to close. Tighten up your whole body: feet, legs, stomach, buttocks, back, shoulders, jaw, face, fists. Hold it . . . Then let it go, all at once. Take a slow deep breath and let it out with a sigh of relief, "Haaaaaa" . . . Relax and let go.

Now just tighten your jaw . . . Does this feel familiar? Does it remind you of any tense situations? Feel the jaw muscles with the fingertips of one hand, just in front of your ears . . . Open and close your mouth a couple of times and notice the movements of these muscles . . . Inhale, exhale, and consciously let your jaw go loose . . . Feel it with your fingertips . . . Imagine a feeling of heaviness in your jaw . . . Let your arms return to a resting position . . . Now raise your shoulders; hold and feel the tension . . . As you let go, exhale and imagine a sense of heaviness in your shoulders.

Now inhale and cup your hands, placing them over your mouth and nose . . . Exhale gently and slowly, and feel the *flowing* of the warm air; imagine it's streaming down your arms and out your fingertips. Do this for two or three breaths. Now allow your arms to relax in a resting position; let them just stay relaxed . . . With the next exhalation, imagine the flowing warmth down your arms and out your fingertips . . . Continue with this image for the next few breaths.

Mentally scan your body, playing "body detective" and looking for those places where you usually experience muscle tension. Briefly tighten any area that feels tense, then let it go . . . Breathe easily and imagine feelings of heaviness throughout your whole body . . . Allow your chest and abdomen to relax more and more as you breathe slower and slower . . . Feel your abdomen expanding outward as you inhale and filling with air . . . Give yourself plenty of time; let the breath move easily in and out at your own pace . . . If any thoughts or concerns arise, just let go and refocus your attention on your breath . . . You may think of these thoughts as attached to clouds that drift briefly across your consciousness and then away . . . Allow your exhalation to lengthen . . . Repeat your special relaxation cue words for the next minute or so.

Whenever you're ready, inhale very slowly, easily, and deeply into your abdomen, going at your own comfortable rate (which may not be the same rate at which the suggestions to breathe come in this script) . . . Feel how your stomach, hips, and lower back expand outward as you inhale, almost like a balloon filling . . . Feel the movement of your abdomen as you inhale. Then exhale . . . Imagine the breath flowing out through your shoulders, down your arms, and out your hands . . . As you exhale, imagine the relaxation flowing like a gentle warmth through your arms as though they were hollow tubes . . . Feel the warmth flowing out through your fingertips as you repeat to yourself, "My arms are heavy and warm; my arms are heavy and warm" . . . Continue to breathe regularly and slowly . . . For the next few minutes feel the movement of breath deep in your abdomen while letting the air flow down your arms with each exhalation . . . Become aware of gentle pulsations, tingling in your fingers, or whatever else you may sense.

And now as you feel your breath deep and slow, imagine you have breathing holes in the bottoms of your feet . . . Imagine the air flowing through your feet as you inhale, coming up through your ankles, knees, and thighs, filling your abdomen slowly and gently. As you exhale, imagine the warm air flowing from your abdomen through your legs and out of your feet and carrying away any remaining tension . . . Breathe in this way for a few moments, while you repeat to yourself, "My legs are heavy and warm; my legs are heavy and warm."

Imagine your blood vessels widening, dilating, as your heart pumps the warm blood down your arms into your hands and through your whole body into your abdomen, legs, and feet. Imagine the warm pink glow of each finger and toe as your blood pulsates through your arterioles, bringing warmth, oxygen, nutrients, and healing to each cell . . . Stay with this image as long as you like, and add other details to it if you wish, picturing and feeling the subtle pulsations. And now imagine the space inside each finger and the space around each finger . . . Feel the peace and quietness.

When you are ready, take a deep breath, gently stretch your body, and open your eyes. Then observe your temperature. If the thermometer is taped on, you can record it instantly. Otherwise, hold the temperature device between the thumb and index finger, wait for one minute while you continue to feel the warmth sensations flowing down the arms and hands, and then record your "POST" temperature on the log sheet.

Each day after you have gone through the script, complete **Log Sheet: Practice 6**. In addition, your log sheets for the next two weeks include questions about the QR practice as well as about Dynamic Relaxation. At the end of the week answer **Questions: Practice 6**. Meet with your group and complete **Discussion and Conclusions: Practice 6**.

Name _____ Date _____

Log Sheet   Quick and Warm: Practice 6

I. After each practice describe (a) the practice situation (your mood, the place, your physical position, etc.), (b) your physical and emotional experiences both during and directly following your practice, and (c) your "Pre" and "Post" hand temperature.

II. Also briefly describe your emotional and physical experiences before, during, and immediately after practicing the Quieting Response (QR) at least two times each day.

III. Describe your cues for stress. These are the inner and outer cues you use as reminders to do QR (e.g., a ringing phone, a tightness in your jaw, a craving for a cigarette or snack).

I.

Day 1   a. _____

Date _____   _____

_____

b. _____

_____

_____

_____

c. Temperature: Pre _____ Post _____

II. QR   _____

experiences   _____

_____

_____

III. Cues   _____

for stress   _____

Day 2   a. _____

Date _____   _____

_____

b. _____

_____

_____

c. Temperature: Pre _____ Post _____

II. QR   _____

experiences   _____

_____

_____

III. Cues   _____

for stress   _____

Day 3   a. _____

Date _____   _____

_____

b. _____

_____

_____

c. Temperature: Pre _____ Post _____

II. QR   _____

experiences   _____

_____

_____

III. Cues   _____

for stress   _____

Day 4   a. _____

Date _____   _____

_____

b. _____

_____

_____

     c. Temperature: Pre _____ Post _____

II. QR   _____

experiences   _____

_____

_____

III. Cues   _____

for stress   _____

Day 5   a. _____

Date _____   _____

_____

     b. _____

_____

_____

     c. Temperature: Pre _____ Post _____

II. QR   _____

experiences   _____

_____

_____

III. Cues   _____

for stress   _____

Day 6   a. _____

Date _____   _____

_____

b. _____

_____

_____

_____

          c. Temperature: Pre _____ Post _____

II. QR   _____

experiences   _____

_____

_____

III. Cues   _____

for stress   _____

Day 7   a. _____

Date _____   _____

_____

          b. _____

_____

_____

_____

          c. Temperature: Pre _____ Post _____

II. QR   _____

experiences   _____

_____

_____

Additional comments/questions:

_____

_____

_____

Name _____ Date _____

Questions   Quick and Warm: Practice 6

1. What benefits occurred as a result of your practice?

_____

_____

_____

_____

_____

2. Did your notice any changes in your hand (foot) temperature and/or in your breathing patterns?

_____

_____

_____

_____

_____

3. Describe your experience of QR. In which situations was it the most useful? The least? How did you remind yourself to do it?

_____

_____

_____

_____

4. In what ways has this week's practice of relaxation and QR affected your daily life? What have been some of the benefits?

_____

_____

_____

_____

5. Comments:

_____

_____

_____

Discussion and Conclusions   Quick and Warm: Practice 6

1. What benefits did the group members notice as a result of the practices?

_____

_____

_____

_____

2. Did group members use similar or different techniques to remind themselves to practice QR? Describe them.

_____

_____

_____

_____

3. What were the similarities and differences associated with the cues of stress?

_____

_____

_____

_____

4. What patterns and experiences occurred with hand warming?

_____

_____

_____

_____

5. Topics for which instructor consultation would be helpful:

_____

_____

_____

List your group members: _____   _____

_____   _____   _____

_____   _____   _____

GENERALIZING RELAXATION: PRACTICE 7

I personally learned quicker in the context of movement as opposed to learning differential relaxation while remaining still. The movement gave me more contrasts, thus maximizing my ability to recognize tense states from loose states. I experimented with just how loose I can become and still execute the task.

STUDENT

Generalizing relaxation into daily life requires mindfulness. It means doing quick body scans several times a day to search for muscles that are being tightened unnecessarily, and then letting the tightness go. It means becoming aware of your breathing, noticing if it becomes short or shallow or if you are holding your breath, and then returning to easy breathing. This takes practice and patience with yourself, so start with the simplest things. Often, bracing is embedded in our habitual daily behaviors. For example, driving in traffic we may clench our jaws, hunch up our shoulders, and grip the steering wheel for dear life. This excessive bracing is part of the startle and/or orienting responses that we evoked when we first learned to drive and that we have not yet unlearned.

In order for relaxation training to have the greatest impact in your life. It is necessary to learn to generalize the skills. In other words, while it is valuable to know how to relax and let go in a quiet, private space, it is equally important to be able to relax and let go of unnecessary tension during the activities of daily life. As a step toward learning these skills, this script encourages relaxation during simple movements. With practice you may learn to stay relaxed while performing increasingly complex and stressful tasks, for example, while driving a car in traffic. Athletes, dancers, and other performers use differential relaxation for peak performance. It allows for more fluidity and grace, besides conserving energy, by relaxing all muscles except those needed for the performance.

Suggestions for Generalizing Relaxation

1. Find the place, posture, time, and setting where you *think* you are most relaxed (watching TV in recliner, sitting in bathtub, etc.) and observe where in your body you're still tight; let it go. A few minutes later, check again: Are you still relaxed? How is your breathing?
2. Have as a goal the ability to keep a part of your awareness on your muscles and breathe at all times, even as you go about your other activities.
3. Do simple art work while concentrating on breathing and relaxation. What do you notice about your art work?
4. Be a relaxed role model for your children.
5. Practice letting go of any unnecessary muscle tension while walking. Before you start, visualize yourself staying relaxed during the movement; look for creative ways to allow your walk to be more relaxed. For example, if you carry books or other things in a heavy shoulder bag, try using a backpack. Notice how you breathe while walking. Be aware of your rhythm. Let walking be a kind of moving meditation.

6. Use your cue word and/or any part of your ritual for relaxation to help you let go. For example, while driving in traffic you might loosen your belt a notch or two as a cue to relax.

7. Progress gradually from relaxing during simple, rhythmic activities to relaxing during more complex ones like cooking, shopping, eating, talking with a friend, doing yoga.

8. Do the differential relaxation as a part of any new activity or behavior that you begin at this time. For example, starting a yoga or an aerobic dance class or even beginning to drive a car that's new to you is a perfect time to build in the new relaxation skills. Or if you have a new job, or job assignment, that requires you to walk up and down a flight of stairs, you could decide that every time you do this particular flight of stairs you will practice your generalization skills. This way you will build up an associative process that quickly becomes automatic.

9. Use mental rehearsal. Plan situations where you will release unneeded tension, and visualize which muscles you might need to relax; feel the relaxation. Then check your visualization against the real-life situation. Which other muscles tightened up that you had not anticipated? Revise your imagery and keep practicing with it.

10. Keep a chart or notebook and give yourself a check mark (or a gold star!) each time you remember to generalize relaxation.

11. You might want to set aside one day a week to practice mindfulness of breathing and relaxing muscles. Go about your activities while giving attention to your breathing and your body. Be aware of your breath and body relaxation while conversing with another, washing dishes, driving, and so on. Taking one day a week for mindfulness will gradually extend into greater self-awareness every day.

Generalizing Relaxation Script

For this exercise have a book or magazine near the chair you will be sitting in and have adequate light for reading.

Get comfortable in a sitting position, allow your eyes to close, and let your body relax and rest. For the next few minutes recreate the sensations you have experienced in your previous relaxation practices . . . Relax all over . . . Allow a pleasant heaviness to develop . . . Allow the comfortable sensations of warmth to flow through your entire body . . . and allow yourself to breathe easily and deeply . . . Take a few moments to scan your body for areas of tension and holding and gently release those areas.

Feel your muscles yielding and relaxing all over. Let the contractions loosen . . . Feel more at rest . . . Let your breathing flow freely and easily without any effort . . . Imagine your blood vessels widening as you relax so that circulation increases without strain or effort . . . Feel the pleasant pulsing and throbbing sensations in your fingers.

Enjoy the serenity of being enveloped by restfulness, heaviness, and warmth . . . Nothing can disturb you . . . Feel the inner restfulness deepening and know that as you relax and enjoy these sensations, you will gain a sense of strength and confidence from the inner peacefulness.

With each exhalation think, "I am relaxed" . . . Concentrate on the feelings of calm that accompany that relaxation; surrender to the good feelings all over.

Now think your cue word or phrase. Think about the words and their meaning to you and feel them more and more . . . Just let the words reverberate inside you. Notice the pleasant feelings you associate with them . . . Experience the feelings as you relax more and more.

Colors can be soothing and relaxing. Think of the color blue; experience the soothing sensations . . . Imagine a deep blue flowing outward, a gentle ocean wave just washing outward, carrying away any tension or strain.

Now, imagine yourself as you sit in the chair. Notice any area of lingering tension and let it go . . . Picture yourself raising your right arm and holding it up while you stay quite relaxed. What sensations can you imagine feeling in the arm? . . . Now, actually raise your right arm and hold it up using the minimum muscle tension necessary for the task. Let the rest of your body stay relaxed . . . Feel the slight tension in your right arm . . . Study the contrast in feeling and notice how it differs from the mental image you had formed . . . Now let your right arm fall to your side and relax it further and further, feeling the difference as the tension drains from your arm.

Again visualize, this time picturing yourself raising your left arm and feeling the feelings of tension . . . Now raise your left arm up and hold it with the minimum effort, feeling the tension in that arm as distinct from the relaxation in the rest of your body . . . Continue to breathe . . . Feel the tension. Let your left arm fall to your side; relax your arm further and further . . . Notice the difference between relaxation and tension.

Imagine raising both arms using the minimum of muscle tension. Now raise both arms. Study the tension . . . Where do you feel it? Let both arms fall limply and notice the tension evaporating.

Visualize yourself standing up in a very relaxed way and walking slowly. Notice which of your muscles may tend to tighten up just by imagining this movement . . . Notice how your breathing changed as you imagined yourself moving . . . Breathe, letting go of any tension.

Open your eyes and maintain the relaxed feelings. Let your eyes move lazily around the room, adjusting to the light . . . When you are ready, stand up slowly while exhaling easily and stand with your feet planted firmly on the floor and well apart . . . Breathe, and relax as much as you can . . . Drop your shoulders, loosen your stomach and knees, let your arms hang loosely . . . Relax and stand still for a few minutes.

Begin to walk slowly back and forth. Let your arms swing gently . . . Let go as much as you can while walking . . . Study your body and release any muscle contractions you don't need . . . Be aware of your breathing as you walk.

Stand still again and relax those parts of your body that are not in use—face, scalp, eyes, jaw . . . Have your tongue rest loosely in your mouth. Breathe easily, with your neck, throat, and shoulders fully relaxed and your stomach relaxed . . . Feel the relaxation in your legs as best you can while standing.

Again think of your cue words or phrase. Just think each word and let each word enhance your overall relaxation . . . Develop the feeling of relaxation while standing.

Now sit down again. Relax comfortably and fully, closing your eyes . . . Rapidly go back into that heavy, comfortable feeling all over and feel the good sensations of warmth throughout your entire body . . . Feel an inner restfulness that deepens and gives you inner strength and confidence . . . Feel all the muscles yielding and letting go as you release contractions everywhere . . . Let yourself feel completely at rest, with your breathing coming freely and easily.

Slowly open your eyes and again allow them to adjust to the lighting in the room . . . Pick up your book or magazine and hold it without reading it yet. Just become aware of the muscle tensions involved in holding it and adjust your position as much as you need to in order to let go of unnecessary muscle tensions . . . Now, while keeping your eyes and forehead as relaxed as possible, begin to read . . . Monitor your breathing and muscle tension every few words or so . . . What tensions can you let go of while still having full comprehension? Relax your jaws, lips, and tongue, . . . your neck and shoulders, your abdomen . . . Breathe freely and easily and go back to your reading.

After you have read a page or so, put the reading material aside, close your eyes, and recreate your relaxed feelings . . . Tell yourself, "I can carry relaxation with me throughout the day" . . . When you are ready, take a deep breath, gently stretch your body, and open your eyes.

Each day after you have gone through the script, complete your **Log Sheet: Practice 7.** You will also be asked to describe one situation each day where you generalized the relaxation skill into an activity. At the end of the week answer **Questions: Practice 7.** Then meet with your group and complete **Discussion and Conclusions: Practice 7.**

Name _____ Date _____

Log Sheet   Generalizing Relaxation: Practice 7

1. After each practice describe (a) the practice situation (your mood, the place, your physical position, etc.) and (b) your physical and emotional experiences both during and directly following your practice.
2. Also briefly describe a situation where you generalized the relaxation skill. Describe which muscles you noticed tightening up, and how your experience of the situation changed when you added the relaxation component to the activity.

Day 1   a. _____

Date _____   _____

_____

               b. _____

_____

_____

Generalize: _____

_____

Day 2   a. _____

Date _____   _____

_____

               b. _____

_____

_____

Generalize: _____

_____

Day 3   a. _____

Date _____   _____

_____

               b. _____

_____

_____

Generalize: _____

_____

Day 4   a. _____
Date _____   _____

_____

           b. _____

_____

Generalize: _____

_____

Day 5   a. _____
Date _____   _____

_____

           b. _____

_____

Generalize: _____

_____

Day 6   a. _____
Date _____   _____

_____

           b. _____

_____

Generalize: _____

_____

Day 7   a. _____
Date _____   _____

_____

           b. _____

_____

Generalize: _____

_____

Name _____ Date _____

Questions Generalizing Relaxation: Practice 7

1. What benefits occurred as a result of your practices?
   _____
   _____
   _____
   _____
   _____

2. In what ways did your ability to perform activities while staying relaxed change over the week? How have your experiences while reading and walking changed as a result of the practices?
   _____
   _____
   _____
   _____
   _____

3. In what ways have the practices affected your daily life experiences, and how did your perception of the world around you change?
   _____
   _____
   _____
   _____

4. In which ways were this week's experiences different from those of previous weeks?
   _____
   _____
   _____

5. What problems/challenges occurred and how did you solve them?
   _____
   _____
   _____

Discussion and Conclusions Generalizing Relaxation: Practice 7

1. What benefits did the group members notice as a result of the practices?

_____

_____

_____

_____

_____

2. Were there common situations where group members found it difficult to generalize relaxation?

_____

_____

_____

_____

_____

3. What creative solutions to problems emerged from the group?

_____

_____

_____

_____

_____

4. Topics for which instructor consultation would be helpful:

_____

_____

List your group members: _____ _____

_____ _____ _____

_____ _____ _____

CREATING YOUR OWN RELAXATION: PRACTICE 8

Writing Your Own Script

Go back over your notes on the previous weeks of practice. What were the parts or aspects of these practice scripts that appealed to you the most or helped you relax most easily? For example, if you found that imagery (Developing a Personal Relaxation Image: Practice 4) was especially helpful to you, you might want to incorporate imagery when you write your own script.

Think also about your own particular body and any chronic areas of tension or discomfort. For example, if you are a woman who has painful menstrual cramps (dysmenorrhea), you might want to include a few suggestions and/or images concerning relaxation and warmth in the pelvic area. Or you may hold chronic tension in your shoulder or neck muscles; if so, you can benefit by including in your script extra repetitions of tensing and relaxing these areas. Or you may want more emphasis on breathing.

Optional: Teach the script in Practice 2 or 3 to a friend or family member. What was it like to be the trainer? What did it do for your own commitment level?

After having completed the dynamic relaxation section of this workbook, review your experiences. Write about them as suggested in the section Reflection and Integration: Summarizing Your Experiences in Chapter 1. This process allows an opportunity to reflect and integrate your experience.

First write your own relaxation script on the **Worksheet: Practice 8**. Then practice this script each day for the next week. If appropriate, make changes and adapt the script. Each day, after you have gone through your script, complete **Log Sheet: Practice 8**. In addition, continue to describe one situation each day in which you have generalized the relaxation skill into an activity. At the end of the week, answer **Questions: Practice 8**. Then meet with your group and complete **Discussion and Conclusions: Practice 8**.

Worksheet   Personal Relaxation Script: Practice 8

In the space below write your own relaxation script.

_____

_____

_____

_____

_____

_____

_____

_____

_____

_____

_____

_____

_____

_____

_____

_____

_____

_____

_____

_____

_____

_____

_____

_____

_____

_____

Name_____ Date_____

Log Sheet   Creating Your Own Relaxation: Practice 8

I. After each practice describe (a) the practice situation (your mood, the place, your physical position, etc.), (b) your physical and emotional experiences both during and directly following your practice, and (c) a situation where you generalized the relaxation skill. Describe how your experience of the situation changed when you added the relaxation component to the activity.

Day 1   a. _____
Date _____   _____
           b. _____
_____
_____
           c. _____
_____
_____

Day 2   a. _____
Date _____   _____
           b. _____
_____
_____
           c. _____
_____
_____

Day 3   a. _____
Date _____   _____
           b. _____
_____
_____
           c. _____
_____
_____

Day 4   a. _____
Date _____   _____
              b. _____
_____
_____
              c. _____
_____
_____
Day 5   a. _____
Date _____   _____
              b. _____
_____
_____
              c. _____
_____
_____
Day 6   a. _____
Date _____   _____
              b. _____
_____
_____
              c. _____
_____
_____
Day 7   a. _____
Date _____   _____
              b. _____
_____
_____
              c. _____
_____
_____

Name _____ Date _____

Questions   Creating Your Own Relaxation: Practice 8

1. How did your practice facilitate relaxation and healing?

_____
_____
_____
_____
_____
_____

2. In what ways did you facilitate generalizing the practice into daily life and how would you do it differently next time?

_____
_____
_____
_____
_____

3. Looking back over Week 8, what parts of your script were helpful to you in encouraging relaxation? Were there components that inhibited relaxation? How did you feel about creating your own script? If you were to revise your script, what improvements might you make in light of your week's experience with it?

_____
_____
_____
_____
_____
_____

4. Comments.

_____
_____

Discussion and Conclusions   Creating Your Own Relaxation:
Practice 8

1. How were the benefits gained during the 8 weeks of practice similar or
   different among group members?

   _____

   _____

   _____

   _____

   _____

2. Were there differences among group members in the scripts they developed?
   What creative parts of their scripts would you incorporate in your script?

   _____

   _____

   _____

   _____

   _____

3. Were there parts of your script that encouraged or prohibited relaxation that
   were common among group members?

   _____

   _____

   _____

   _____

   _____

4. Topics for which instructor consultation would be helpful:

   _____

   _____

   _____

List your group members: _____ _____

_____ _____ _____

_____ _____ _____

SUGGESTED READINGS

Bernstein, D. A. & Borkovec, T. D. (1973). *Progressive Relaxation Training: A Manual for the Helping Professions.* Champaign, IL: Research Press.

Fried, R. (1990). *The Breath Connection.* New York: Plenum.

Green, E. E. & Green, A. M. (1977). *Beyond Biofeedback.* New York: Delacorte.

Hanh, T. N. (1976). *The Miracle of Mindfulness! A Manual on Meditation.* Boston: Beacon Press.

Hanna, T. (1988). *Somatics.* Reading, MA: Addison-Wesley.

Jacobson, E. (1974). *Progressive Relaxation* (3rd ed.). Chicago: University of Chicago Press.

Levey, J. & Levey, M. (1987). *The Fine Arts of Relaxation, Concentration and Meditation.* Boston: Wisdom.

Lichstein, K. L. (1988). *Clinical Relaxation Strategies.* New York: Wiley.

Mason, L. J. (1980). *Guide to Stress Reduction.* Culver City, CA: Peace Press.

Parker, S. (1989). *The Lungs and Breathing.* New York: Franklin Watts.

Peper, E. (1990). *Breathing for Health with Biofeedback.* Montreal: Thought Technology.

Peper, E. & Williams, E. A. (1981). *From the Inside Out: A Self-Teaching and Laboratory Manual for Biofeedback.* New York: Plenum.

Rama, S., Ballentine, R., & Hymes, A. (1979). *Science of Breath.* Honesdale, PA: Himalayan International Institute of Yoga Science and Philosophy Publishers.

Stroebel, C. F. (1982). *QR: The Quieting Reflex.* New York: Putnam.

Chapter 3
Cognitive Balance

A human being fashions his consequences as surely as he fashions his goods or his dwelling. Nothing that he says, thinks or does is without consequences.

NORMAN COUSINS

We are what our thoughts have made us; so take care about what you think. Words are secondary. Thoughts live; they travel far.

SWAMI VIVEKANANDA

INTRODUCTION TO COGNITIVE BALANCE

Beware of psychosclerosis: the hardening of the attitudes.

Through the process of learning dynamic relaxation, you may have observed that body tensions are part of mental tensions. The process of somatic relaxation encourages awareness, mindfulness, and passive attention. Thinking patterns are intertwined and part of somatic patterns; this process is more easily observed when you become quiet. When the soma is quiet, the effect of thoughts and feelings can be more easily felt in the body. The content of thoughts can have a dramatic effect on our body tensions; just notice how differently your body feels when thinking about an anger-provoking incident as compared to thinking about a peaceful scene or a lover.

For profound and lasting changes in body tension to take place, usually some rearranging of thinking patterns is necessary. This awareness and changing of thinking patterns we call cognitive balancing. For example, if you are constantly judging your own performance and feeling "not good enough," this thought by itself can create both mental and physical tension. Dynamic relaxation may help to undo some of this tension; however, it will always return whenever such thoughts are present. Hence, we need also to learn to change the thought sequences.

Often, we resist letting go of our dysfunctional and irrational thought patterns since we may use these thoughts to identify ourselves, as, for example, when we say, "I know I can't learn Japanese" or "I am stupid" or "I never let any SOB cut in front of me on the freeway." We may fear that if we changed our patterns, we would have to accept, face, or let go of who we are. Or we may believe that these ways of thinking are necessary for generating our best performances or that it is impossible to change the thought patterns. So often thoughts appear automatically and apparently beyond our control.

Our thoughts often include many hypnotic suggestions from our culture or family that limit our potential. If we become aware of, accept, and change those habitual thinking processes that act as hypnotic inductions, we can expand our health and potential. It is truly amazing to witness the tenacity of a thought pattern. Dr. Deepak Chopra, a well-known Ayurvedic physician, states in his book *Quantum Healing* that our mental patterns are largely responsible for creating our bodies: "memory must be more permanent than matter. What is a cell, then? It is a memory that has built some matter around itself, forming a specific pattern. Your body is just the place your memory calls home."

Life is change and thoughts, even though they may seem permanent, can change as we grow. Yet making changes in habitual thought patterns requires patience with oneself, an experimental attitude, flexibility, openness, and, above all, a sense of humor. Observing and changing our thought patterns to mobilize health are basic approaches of rational emotive therapy (Ellis, 1979) and cognitive–behavioral psychology (Meichenbaum, 1977), as well as components of many meditative practices. The underlying principles of most cognitive therapies are the following:

1. All humans are irrational at times in our assumptions and expectations of the world, self, and others. Most likely, it is delusional to believe that the world can be rationally understood. For example, how do we rationally understand birth, death, love, art, or music?
2. Cognitive activity (thought) affects behavior. We are mainly disturbed by our absolutist beliefs and demands about events rather than by negative events themselves. It is not the events that disturb us, it is our perception of those events: The sound of footsteps can evoke fear, if it is late at night on the street, or pleasant expectancy, if we are anticipating the approach of a loved one.
3. Distorted thinking patterns can be observed, challenged, and transcended. We can change our demands to preferences, using cognitive and behavior change methods. Desired behavior change will be effected through cognitive change.

Our thoughts, or cognitions, are often similar to a pair of glasses, or contact lenses, through which we perceive reality. They are so close to us that we are usually not aware of the possible distortion. Do we see through rose-colored glasses or charcoal-tinted ones? Another way to say this is that we are constantly bombarded by sensory inputs and must learn to interpret and filter out a large portion of them so that we can create a sense of order and meaning. We tend to let in those experiences that support our belief systems and discard the rest because we hate to be wrong and would often rather be "right" even if it makes us miserable. We often focus on negative experiences and disregard positive ones in order to support our beliefs which may be generalizations like "The world is a dangerous place," "Men are no good," or "This government serves only the rich."

Thus, our emotional distress may be due less to an event than to our interpretation of it.

How do our thoughts distort reality? Depression and anxiety are often due to a negative view of oneself, the world, and/or the future (e.g., "There is no hope . . . I failed the exam; now I won't be able to graduate. No one will hire me"). By replacing maladaptive or irrational *automatic thoughts* with more rational, positive ones and by identifying and questioning underlying negative beliefs, many people can overcome depression and anxiety. The events and circumstances in our lives may not change, but as our perceptions and beliefs become less distorted, our emotional experiences improve.

Perhaps language is the most important means of shaping and structuring our perception of reality. How we experience reality is determined, in large part, by how we talk to ourselves about it. This is one reason why talking about our troubles, or even writing about them, can be so helpful in understanding and integrating our experience. Putting events and emotional responses into language (by speaking or writing) seems to provide distance, perspective, and structure on what would otherwise be overwhelming and chaotic. Even keeping log notes helps build the "witness" part of us, which observes without emotional attachment.

When we listen in to our automatic inner language, it may also become easier to identify any distortions and shift them. In addition, we can learn to say useful things to ourselves (self-instructions). For example, if we are about to give a speech, we can say to ourselves, "The audience will be attentive. I am breathing slowly; I can smile and relax." Simply substituting "I choose" for "I have to" can change our experience. This inner language is not only the overt phrases and statements we use; it is often the background worrying that continues as we are doing other things. So often we are only partially present while performing specific tasks. A large part of us is ruminating. How much more potential we could activate if we channel that "worry energy" used in the rumination into performance of the task at hand.

The language we use both creates and describes our images. Hence, imagery is an important tool for changing thoughts. Going over a mistake strengthens the chance of repeating it; imaging success builds a better performance. A form of mental rehearsal is used to help improve performance on an exam or in music or sports. It is often used in systematic desensitization to help people overcome phobias. For example, a person who fears snakes learns to relax. Then he imagines, by stages, getting closer and closer to the snake without fear. When he can imagine relaxing while holding a snake, the final step will be a structured, safe, real-world experience with a snake.

So often we are covertly conditioned to respond to stimuli outside and inside ourselves. The cognitive balance process allows us to increase our freedom through reducing automatic, conditioned thought patterns. Instead of getting our buttons pushed by events, we can take control by observing and changing our inner dialogue about those events. The inner dialogue, made up of cultural and familial injunctions that have held us with hypnotic power, can be transformed into a positive tool for self-change. Expressing our secrets (through writing) can be another way to dissolve those constraining injunctions, thus freeing more of our intrinsic potential.

Finally, our patterns of thinking about illness are shaped by strong cultural and family traditions. Many of us learned early on that getting sick was a guilt-free way to avoid obligations, such as school or social gatherings, as well as to receive extra care and attention. Such rewards can reinforce the pattern of getting sick. The "shoulds," "oughts," and "musts" of our cultural and familial conditioning are so strong that often it takes an illness to allow us the freedom to put them aside. Why not learn to challenge these constraints so that we can get our needs met without having to get sick? By exploring the advantages of illness, we can develop alternative approaches to getting needs met without having to become ill.

CHANGING THE INTERNAL DIALOGUE: PRACTICE 9

We are formed and molded by our thoughts. Those whose minds are shaped by selfless thoughts give joy when they speak or act. Joy follows them like a shadow that never leaves them.

THE BUDDHA

Life consists in what a man is thinking of all day.

RALPH WALDO EMERSON

I took a different attitude toward my illness. . . . I looked at it as necessary or as a learning experience and refused to say things to myself such as "I am never going to get better". . . . I got better faster than usual. I feel that this was due in part to controlling the panic I usually feel when I get sick during the school year.

STUDENT

I approached illness in a nonjudgmental, welcoming way, seeing symptoms as messages to be understood, not suppressed. I found that blame-free language helped me to eliminate my guilt, too.

STUDENT

Sometimes our internal language (self-talk) is the main place where words like *should* and *can't* appear. Does your internal dialogue empower or undermine you? Do you perceive yourself as a helpless victim, boxed into a set of obligations and struggling to be barely acceptable, or as a powerful person with many choices? Every time we say, "I should," we make ourselves wrong or not good enough. As you rewrite your self-talk, you will be rebuilding your self-esteem.

Reframing

Reframing, a term used in neurolinguistic programming, means the process of voluntarily shifting perception, usually from a negative image to a more positive one, for example, from powerlessness to choice, from threat to challenge, from nuisance to blessing in disguise. It can also refer to revising a memory of the past in order to correct a mistake.

In studies done by Kobasa, Maddi, and Kahn (1982), people who coped well with stress and stayed healthy were compared with others in similar situations who became ill. The researchers identified three characteristics of the "hardy" personality: commitment (rather than alienation), sense of control (rather than helplessness), and viewing change as challenge (rather than threat). This means that a large part of coping is how we "frame" (or talk to ourselves about) our experience. For example, in doing dynamic relaxation practice "powerless" self-talk would be, "I have to (should, ought to) do my dynamic relaxation practice"; "choice/control" self-talk would be, "I deserve to have a break; I choose to do dynamic relaxation" or "I have the opportunity to do dynamic relaxation."

As another example, suppose everyone you live and work with has been coming down with colds or the flu. "Threat" self-talk would be, "I always catch everything that's going around" or "I know I'll be next; I can't avoid it." On the other hand, "challenge" self-talk would be, "In the past I might have caught that bug. Now, I will build up my immune system with extra rest, eating well, drinking more fluids, more vitamin C, and I'll stay healthy."

Our feelings of helplessness can easily shift to feelings of strength and re-sourcefulness if we reframe the situation. For example, a young boy with migraines was reluctant to practice his hand-warming skills at home. When his therapist asked him if he would be willing to help make a video in order to show other children how to learn to warm their hands, the boy practiced with great enthusiasm in order to be a movie star. Similarly, a nursing instructor who had a multicultural group of students felt upset by their behavior, which she felt was rude and disrespectful at times. Deciding she could write a book about strategies other teachers could use for teaching culturally diverse students offered her a new viewpoint. Now she could experiment with new teaching strategies in order to become an expert and have something valuable to share with others. To learn more about her students was no longer just a way of helping herself but a way of making a contribution to others in her profession.

Einstein once remarked that the most important question we must each answer for ourselves is "Is the universe a friendly place?" If your answer is yes, then even seeming catastrophes can be viewed as opportunities or challenges. Bernie Siegel, a well-known surgeon who works with cancer patients to enable their self-healing, illustrates this point with the following story: A man is on his way to the airport, rushing to make the plane, when he has a flat tire. Imagine his feelings as he sweats and struggles to put the spare on; anger at himself for not leaving earlier, anger at the tire, anger at the whole world. When he finally arrives, his plane has just taken off. In disgust, he drives home, flipping the radio on for a bit of distraction. On the news he hears that the plane he missed has just crashed shortly after takeoff. He kisses the flat tire!

Is it possible that the things you thought were a nuisance or a curse could turn out, when viewed from a broad enough perspective, to be a gift or blessing? "To accept the things we cannot change," as in the Alcoholics Anonymous Serenity Prayer, does not mean passivity or resignation but something closer to trusting that while we do our best to deal with what *is* within our power to change, all will be well.

The language we use often reflects how we feel about ourselves and how honestly we are willing to communicate with others. Such common phrases as "but," "I should," and "I can't" may be replaced with phrases that reflect a greater degree of self-confidence and/or honesty. Martin Seligman (1991), a well-known psychologist at the University of Pennsylvania, has codified explanatory styles into three categories. The following is a brief outline of his concept of internal language and learned optimism[1]:

1. *Stable versus unstable* language describes an experience as a permanent versus a transient situation (e.g., "It's *always* this way").
2. *Global versus specific* language describes an experience as affecting the person's entire life versus affecting a specific aspect of his or her life (e.g., "It's the story of my life").
3. *Internal versus external* language describes a situation as being caused by the person versus being caused at least in part by the situation or circumstances (e.g., "It's all my fault"). A systems approach assumes that all phenomena are interdependent; thus, there is a balance between personal responsibility and the system in which we are embedded.

The distinctions in these explanatory styles have important health implications. Somatic and psychological symptoms of helplessness and depression may be correlated with stable, global, and internal explanatory styles for negative events. (In animal studies, Visintainer, Volpicelli, and Seligman, 1982, showed that rats that were conditioned to experience helplessness were more likely to develop cancer and die than rats that were not similarly conditioned.) The following suggestions may be used to guide you in your practice this week:

1. *Shift "always" to "at this time."* Instead of saying, "I always make mistakes on exams," say, "I have made mistakes in the past on exams" or "I am making mistakes today on this exam." This does not imply that you will always make mistakes in the future on exams. Absolute statements have a self-hynotic effect. The first step in changing self-image and internal dialogue is to change the way we describe ourselves and our past experiences to others. This leaves the door open for change. Otherwise, because we don't want to break our predictions, we will stay stuck.
2. *Change "I can't" to "I haven't taken the time to learn to." or "I haven't chosen to learn to."* "I can't ski" can be changed to "I have not chosen to take the time to learn how to ski." Sometimes "I can't" may really mean "I prefer not to" or "At this time I don't see a way to."
3. *Change "should" to "choose" or "choose not."* This language change implies assertiveness rather than passivity or aggressiveness. "I should do my home practice" becomes "I choose to do my home practice." The attitude and expectancy of rewards are different in these two statements. "I could" also implies choices. Sometimes the "should" is stated as "I have to"; this

too can be rephrased using "choose" or "could." When you hear yourself saying, "I have to," you might also try substituting "I get to," as in "I get to dress up for the party."

4. *Change "but" to "and."* When you say, "I really like your new haircut, but it could be a little longer," what you are really saying is that you don't like their new haircut because it's too short. If you say, "I really like your new haircut, and it could be a little longer," you are communicating that you are used to their hair longer and you like it that way and you also like it the way it is cut now. Of course, another option is that you may not actually like their new haircut at all. You may choose to say nothing about the new haircut rather than to criticize it.

5. *Change absolute statements to relative statements.* This suggestion relates to our conceptual framework rather than to specific words or phrases. For example, during a standoff in an argument with his spouse, a man at first thought, "We're stuck," which meant to him that there was no hope for change. He then reframed this to "We are pausing," which implied that the disagreement would be resolved. Another example: "I am an asthmatic" can be changed to "On certain occasions, I wheeze."

6. *It is important to avoid rehearsing a bad experience in your mind as you think about it or retell it.* This concept is used by professional athletes. For example, one of the authors asked a professional world-class skeet shooter what she does when she misses. She replied that she assesses what she did wrong, sees herself correcting the mistake, and then pictures herself doing it again in her mind perfectly. That way she never rehearses the mistake again.

Choosing New Phrases

Be aware of your language. Whenever you think, intend to speak, or actually speak, change self-defeating words and phrases to self-enhancing ones:

From	To
but. . .	and. . .
I can't. . .	I haven't taken the time to learn to. . .
	I prefer not to. . .
I have to. . .	I will or I want to. . .
I should. . .	I choose or I could. . .
I'm afraid to. . .	I'm afraid to and I'll do it anyway. . .
	I want to. . .
	I am excited about. . .
I never. . .	I seldom. . .
I always. . .	I sometimes/often. . .

Written Exercise

To practice changing your habitual self-statements, write out your old state-ment and then substitute a new empowering phrase. On the **Worksheet: Changing the Internal Dialogue: Practice 9** complete the sentence with your most habitual thoughts or statement. Then, say the empowering sentences to yourself (or to a partner) and notice the effect it has on you (and/or your partner).

Optional: With a partner practice using positive phrases while talking about topics in which have to, should, and must are typically used, such as in areas of obligation. The partner who is the listener makes a note on paper each time a negative phrase is accidentally used and gives feedback after a few minutes. Then partners reverse roles.

Ask friends and family members to help you become aware of your use of these phrases. Agree with a friend to monitor each other's use of but, should, can't, etc., for one week. The one who uses these words most takes the other to dinner.

Tape-record your own conversation, then play it back and listen to how you speak. Each time you observe yourself using limiting phrases, restate them and speak them out loud.

The objectives of this home practice are the following:

1. To increase awareness of language patterns
2. To develop the ability to change these patterns
3. To observe the effects of these changes

During the week whenever you think, intend to speak, or actually speak, monitor your language and immediately substitute an empowering phrase when-ever possible. Each day complete **Log Sheet: Practice 9.** At the end of the week answer **Questions: Practice 9.** Meet with your group and complete **Discussion and Conclusions: Practice 9.**

Name _____ Date _____

Worksheet   Changing the Internal Dialogue: Practice 9

1. I should _____

_____

_____

Empowering phrase: _____

_____

_____

2. I have to _____

_____

_____

Empowering phrase: _____

_____

_____

3. I should have _____

_____

_____

Empowering phrase: _____

_____

_____

4. I can't _____

_____

_____

Empowering phrase: _____

_____

_____

5. I'm afraid to _____

_____

_____

Empowering phrase: _____

_____

_____

6. I always _____

_____

_____

Empowering phrase: _____

_____

_____

7. I never _____

_____

_____

Empowering phrase: _____

_____

_____

Name _____ Date _____

Log Sheet Changing the Internal Dialogue: Practice 9

Each day note (a) How easy was it for you to notice your use of the *old* phrases. (b) Describe situations (your emotional state, the presence of others, etc.) when it was easy or difficult for you to be aware of and use the *new* phrases. (c) What did you experience when you used the new phrases?

Day 1   a. _____
Date _____   _____

_____

            b. _____

_____

            c. _____

_____

Day 2   a. _____
Date _____   _____

_____

            b. _____

_____

            c. _____

_____

Day 3   a. _____
Date _____   _____

_____

            b. _____

_____

            c. _____

_____

Day 4   a. _____
Date _____   _____
                  _____
               b. _____
                  _____
               c. _____
                  _____

Day 5   a. _____
Date _____   _____
                  _____
               b. _____
                  _____
               c. _____
                  _____

Day 6   a. _____
Date _____   _____
                  _____
               b. _____
                  _____
               c. _____
                  _____

Day 7   a. _____
Date _____   _____
                  _____
               b. _____
                  _____
               c. _____
                  _____

Questions   Changing the Internal Dialogue: Practice 9

1. What benefits occurred as a result of your practices?

_____

_____

_____

_____

2. Describe common situations where it was easy or difficult to be aware of and substitute the new phrases.

_____

_____

_____

_____

3. Describe the process in which you intercepted the limiting phrases and substituted the empowering ones. How often were you able to choose the empowering phrase before speaking it?

_____

_____

_____

_____

4. How did changing your language change your experience of yourself and/or the world?

_____

_____

_____

5. What problems/challenges, if any, occurred?

_____

_____

_____

_____

Discussion and Conclusions Changing the Internal Dialogue: Practice 9

1. What benefits did the group members notice as a result of the practice?

_____
_____
_____
_____
_____
_____

2. Describe common situations where it was easy or difficult to be aware of and substitute the new phrases.

_____
_____
_____
_____
_____

3. How did the experience of substituting empowering phrases instead of the habitual ones differ among group members?

_____
_____
_____
_____
_____

4. Topics for which instructor consultation would be helpful:

_____
_____

List your group members: _____ _____

_____ _____ _____

_____ _____ _____

TRANSFORMING FAILURE INTO SUCCESS: PRACTICE 10

During the slalom race, I was going too fast. I was thrown by a bump and exploded on the slope at fifty miles per hour. The ski patrol got me, put me in the toboggan, and took me down the slope and then to the hospital. All the time I was asking why and how come this happened. Every time someone came to visit, they again asked, "What happened? How did you get injured?" Each time I recited the accident.

Finally, when I got back to competitive skiing, I had lost the edge. Each time I went fast or hit a bump, I got scared and felt just like I did when I was injured. Then I realized that I had rehearsed how to ski with failure. I had rehearsed the accident scene hundreds of times. First when I kept asking why, and then when I retold the event to my coach, parents, friends, and anyone who asked. I had overlearned the bad habit of stiffening whenever I was going fast.

Once I realized this, I asked myself, "How could I have skied differently so that I would not have been hurt?" The answer was obvious: The moment I was going too fast, I would have exhaled, flexed my knees, and retracted my legs as I hit the bump. Then I would have slowed down. At this point, I started to rehearse this new image. In fact, every time I thought of skiing or the accident, I imaged this new scene. I continued this process even when friends asked me about my accident. Instead of telling them about it, I now answered, "I got injured, and let me tell you how I would ski it now."

After practicing this for a few weeks, my skiing improved remarkably. It taught me an important lesson. Instead of going over failure, I now ask, "What can I learn from it? How would I do this differently?" I now spend my time rehearsing how I would like to do it, instead of how not to do it.

What we think about and rehearse is the template for future actions. Our past rehearsal prepares us for future action. We all stumble, make mistakes, and repeat old negative behavior patterns that do not work for us, but we can change the thoughts and images of failure into successful learning moments to create a successful future, a major process of changing our future behavior. Through changing our previous self-defeating or limiting patterns we can correct our errors and thereby learn from the past. Mistakes and errors are feedback, and feedback is essential for growth. Therefore errors, mistakes, or wrongdoings are *opportunities* to learn from. When we think about the past event, we need not remember how it actually happened, since that would just encourage the same pattern to occur again. Instead, we can image how we could have done it differently, thereby creating a new template for future action. Remember, making mistakes is not a bad thing; in fact, it is the major source of learning. However, *repeating* mistakes is a waste of time.

What happens when we act foolishly, make a mistake, or get into a fight? Often, we look back and feel guilty or bad about ourselves. We may try to analyze and ask why the behavior occurred. Perhaps we use the image of failure to beat ourselves up, repeatedly chastising ourselves for what we did: "I shouldn't have done . . ." or "I can never seem to . . ." We may even believe that this process of reminding ourselves again and again of not doing the wrong thing is a good strategy to *make sure it won't happen again.* Unfortunately, this strategy of reminding yourself of what not to do only strengthens the memory of the mistake since you mentally rehearse it each time you think of not doing it. Hence, what is frequently rehearsed is more likely to be repeated.

The alternative is simple: *Learn from your mistakes.* Ask: "With the wisdom I now have, how could I do things differently in that situation?" We can all play Monday morning quarterback since hindsight is 20/20. This means that we have the wisdom and resources to change and not repeat our mistakes. When you notice yourself thinking, "I wish I'd done that differently," stop. Give yourself credit for being aware of the thought. Breathe and relax, then ask yourself, "If I could do this over, what would I do?" Then imagine yourself doing it in the new way.

Whenever we visualize or mentally rehearse in our minds, we are strengthening behaviors. We are reinforcing engrams. Engrams are well-established pathways in the nervous system along which information flows, making certain thoughts and behaviors habitual. In the process of conditioning there appears to be no difference between actual rehearsal and imagined rehearsal; both strengthen the engram. The rehearsed behavior then occurs, which in turn reinforces the mental pattern. The major question is: Which pattern would you like to reinforce?

We consciously or unconsciously mentally rehearse so that our real lives will go more smoothly. For example, you may anticipate questions that might be asked at a meeting. As you think of the questions, you also practice the answers. In a more structured form, you may at some time have done "role playing," such as pretending that your friend is a prospective employer who is interviewing you for a job; you practiced how you would introduce yourself and even the responses you wanted to give. Role rehearsal makes the actual behavior much easier, especially if you do it a few times; in the role playing you are reinforcing a desirable behavior. Most, if not all, politicians, from the president downward, role rehearse their answers to possible questions to be asked at a press conference before they actually have the press conference; it's no wonder that they appear to proceed so smoothly.

Mental rehearsal is role playing done in your imagination. The more you imagine yourself performing the desired behavior, the more likely it is that you will actually perform that behavior. Almost all athletes and performers mentally rehearse their performance as the major tool in enhancing their optimal performance. This is illustrated by the golfer who miscalculated at the fourth hole and hit the ball into the pond. Instead of cursing himself and feeling dumb, the wise golfer acknowledged that a mistake occurred and then asked himself, "What was the problem?" He then considered that he might not have hit the ball hard enough or that he might not have accounted for the crosswind—or that he did not know and needed to ask a consultant for suggestions. He decided that he had not accounted for the crosswinds and then asked, "How could I have done it differently to get the outcome I wanted?" He then imagined exactly how hard and in what direction to hit the ball. He mentally rehearsed the appropriate swing a number of times, each time seeing the ball landing on the green just a short putt away from the fifth hole. As he imaged this perfect swing, he felt it in his body. A bit later when his golfing partner asked him what happened when his ball went into the pond, he answered, "It went into the pond, and let me tell you how I would hit it now." Thus, the past error became the cue to rehearse the desired behavior. To make the mental rehearsal even more useful, the golfer could continue this practice after every swing. In addition, he might imagine a slightly different situation coming up in the future and imagine himself performing perfectly in that situation also. For example, he might imagine that he will be confronted by a large sand trap; again, he calculates the force necessary to clear the obstacle, feels himself doing it perfectly, and watches the ball sail across to the green on the other side.

We all have more wisdom and resources at our command when we are relaxed and in a positive frame of mind. Mental rehearsal gives us an opportunity to take charge and change situations in which we have made mistakes. It is a process of accepting what is and what happened without blaming, judging, or criticizing ourselves. The past memory of the personal failure or poor coping behavior becomes an opportunity and trigger to imagine ourselves acting more wisely, compassionately, or in whatever manner we would prefer. Thus, we rehearse and strengthen the desirable behavior.

Consider the problem behavior of overeating, especially at parties. Often, would-be dieters look back with chagrin on how they wolfed down cookies and cakes. They conclude that they have no will power, which makes them feel bad about themselves. The internal language is something like, "I shouldn't have eaten that stuff—the shrimp toasties, the egg rolls, the chocolate mousse; I can never control myself at parties." If you are an overeater, try an alternative approach instead of self-blame and continued mental rehearsal of eating the wrong things. Visualize yourself first relaxing at the party by doing QR, then picking up a handful of baby carrots, slowly chewing each one and tasting its sweetness, and then drinking a sparkling soda water with a twist of lemon.

Similarly, if your goal includes more exercise, do you find yourself saying, "I shouldn't have watched TV yesterday" or "I'm such a lazy bum"? Guilt does not produce the results you want. Instead, say, "I choose to run" and visualize yourself first walking to the TV to turn it off, then turning away from it, putting your running shoes on, heading out the door, breathing in the cool air, and feeling invigorated.

To practice rewriting the past, it is best to begin with relatively easy things. For example, suppose you are often impatient when waiting in long lines; the last time that happened you felt yourself becoming annoyed, tense, and angry. When you reached the checkout clerk, who seemed to be very slow, you growled and gave her a dirty look. Now you have decided that you would like to behave differently, that it is not helpful to get upset over such an event. Imagine yourself again in the long line, feeling the first feelings of irritation; then remember your decision and say, "This is silly." Next, take a deep breath and relax, realizing that this is a lovely opportunity to let go. As the clerk begins your order, say to him: "It sure must be a drag to have such long lines." As you leave, congratulate yourself for the ease with which you kept control and for being kind to the clerk.

General Guidelines

Image in total detail: see and feel the experience. Imagine every small step, sensation, and thought—everything that would occur when you actually do the task. How you image the task is not important. Some people see it in living color while others have only a sense of it. Just take yourself through the new activity. Rewriting the past takes practice. During the mental rehearsal the old pattern often reasserts itself. Just let it go and practice again. If it continues to recur, ask yourself, "What do I need to learn from this; what is my lesson?"

You can only change yourself. Remember that others have the freedom and the right to react in their own way. In your imagery, see yourself changing. Others may also change in their response to your change; however, they have the right NOT to change.

Specific Instructions

Begin by thinking of a past behavior you would like to change. Write out your new behavior pattern, using the wisdom you now have, on **Worksheet: Behavior Rewrite: Practice 10.** Then practice the **Transforming Success into Failure Script.** During the visualization, you might elaborate upon or even change your new pattern. Finally, once during the day observe an action you experience as an error (however small) and at that moment mentally rewrite how you would like to have behaved. Use the following five-step process:

1. Think of a past conflict or area of behavior with which you are dissatisfied.
2. Ask, "How could I have done this differently?"
3. See yourself in that same situation but behaving differently, using the wisdom you now have (you might want to rehearse this step a number of times).
4. Picture a possible future situation where you could react in the old pattern and see yourself doing it differently, using the desired behavior.
5. Smile and congratulate yourself for taking charge of programming your own future.

Remember, you will *really* strengthen your new behavior pattern when you also practice it in real life!

Optional: Find a partner to do this with. Then, think of a time when you acted in a way you would now like to change. Mentally rehearse the new strategy. Then share your new behavior strategy as if it really had *happened; that is, describe to your partner not the actual event that happened but how you wish you had behaved—as if the desired behavior had actually occurred in the past.*

Repeat the exercise by switching roles.

Notice to what extent you still want to explain what actually happened versus truly allowing the new pattern to be presented as if it had already taken place in the past.

Before beginning the **Transforming Failure into Success Script,** take some time to write out the new behavior pattern that you would like to rehearse on **Worksheet: Behavior Rewrite: Practice 10.**

Name _____ Date _____

Worksheet   Behavior Rewrite: Practice 10

Behavior to rewrite: _____
_____
_____

Detailed description of new behavior pattern: _____
_____
_____
_____
_____
_____
_____
_____
_____
_____
_____
_____
_____
_____
_____
_____
_____
_____
_____
_____
_____
_____
_____
_____

Transforming Failure into Success Script

Get into a comfortable position. Tighten all the muscles in your body; feel the tension... Let go and relax; feel the relaxation spreading... Let your eyes be closed... Focus on your breathing, letting it become very relaxed, very low in your abdomen... Allow your abdomen to expand with your breath as you inhale; feel your pelvis widening... Exhale and feel the tension leaving your body as your abdomen comes in... Let the breathing be slow and effortless... As you exhale, imagine a blue wave going out further and further... Let the relaxation deepen as your breathing deepens, allowing yourself to sink into a pleasant relaxed state... Use your cue words to deepen your relaxation.

Allow the memory of the past event in which you would like to have acted differently to come into your mind now... Observe it from beginning to end from a detached viewpoint, as if watching a movie... Ask yourself, "Given the wisdom I have now, how might I have behaved differently?"... Examine your options; there may be many different ways of responding... Let the answers and images flow into your awareness, or use the previously written desired pattern.

Now go back to the behavior you would like to rewrite. See yourself in it once again, only this time go through it in a new way... Rerun the movie, imagining the event, the people, and the whole situation in detail, except this time see and feel yourself behaving in the new way... See yourself acting with confidence and control, breathing comfortably and easily the whole time... Remember, you cannot change others; the only person you have control over is yourself. See how others respond to your new behavior.

When you have finished reliving the scene, focus on your breathing; feel the widening and narrowing of your abdomen as you inhale and exhale... Allow the feelings of relaxation and peacefulness to be present.

Now either repeat the scene once more or picture a similar situation that could occur in the future. See and feel yourself behaving with the new pattern.

When you have finished experiencing this scene, return to your slow, easy breathing... Feel the peacefulness and calm; let the relaxation occur as your breathing slows. Let your exhalation lengthen... Be aware of the change in feelings about the event. Note the sense of control and autonomy... Enjoy the feelings and remember that the more you mentally practice, the more likely it is that you will achieve the desired outcome... Then take a deep breath, stretch, gently open your eyes, and feel peacefully alert.

Each day after you have gone through the script, complete **Log Sheet: Practice 10.** At the end of the week answer **Questions: Practice 10.** Meet with your group and complete **Discussion and Conclusions: Practice 10.**

Log Sheet Transforming Failure into Success: Practice 10

1. After each practice describe the experience of rewriting your past in your imagination while being relaxed (you may use the same or a different event each day).
2. Each day describe one situation or experience that you chose to rewrite mentally. Do this right after the occurrence of the event. Describe how it changed your feelings about the event.

Day 1   1. _____

Date _____   _____

_____

            2. _____

_____

_____

_____

Day 2   1. _____

Date _____   _____

_____

            2. _____

_____

_____

_____

Day 3   1. _____

Date _____   _____

_____

            2. _____

_____

_____

_____

Day 4   1. _____
Date _____   _____

_____

    2. _____

_____

_____

_____

Day 5   1. _____
Date _____   _____

_____

    2. _____

_____

_____

_____

Day 6   1. _____
Date _____   _____

_____

    2. _____

_____

_____

_____

Day 7   1. _____
Date _____   _____

_____

    2. _____

_____

_____

_____

Additional comments/questions:

_____

_____

138

Name_____ Date_____

Questions Transforming Failure into Success: Practice 10

1. What benefits occurred as a result of your practices?

_____
_____
_____
_____
_____

2. How did your feelings change?

_____
_____
_____
_____
_____

3. How might this practice affect your reaction in future events?

_____
_____
_____
_____
_____

4. What problems/challenges occurred and how did you solve them?

_____
_____
_____
_____
_____

Discussion and Conclusions Transforming Failure into Success:
Practice 10

1. What benefits did the group members notice as a result of the practice?

_____

_____

_____

_____

_____

_____

2. Describe common themes that the group members chose to rewrite.

_____

_____

_____

_____

_____

_____

3. Among group members, how were the experiences of this week's practice
related to ease of the practice, and belief in the efficacy of mental rehearsal?

_____

_____

_____

_____

_____

_____

4. Topics for which instructor consultation would be helpful:

_____

_____

List your group members: _____ _____

_____ _____ _____

_____ _____ _____

FREEING THE HIDDEN SECRETS: PRACTICE 11[2]

A human being has so many skins inside, covering the depths of the heart. We know so many things, but we don't know ourselves! Why, thirty or forty skins or hides, as thick and hard as an ox's or a bear's, cover the soul. Go into your own ground and learn to know yourself there.

MEISTER ECKHART

I wanted to tell my girlfriend that my father was crazy, yet I could not. Would she suspect me? What would she think? How could I talk about the shame in my family? I can tell no one. I can't even talk to my family. Definitely not my father; he just drifts away. Not my mother; she just does not want to hear it.

I must keep it a secret so no one will know. The myth of my perfect family must continue at any cost. Yet, how can I be truly close to my girlfriend, if I can not share my life? Each time I talk I have to edit, I block, I pull a curtain down, I tighten up.

STUDENT

We are inhibited whenever we keep secrets or don't express our true thoughts and feelings about an emotionally upsetting experience in our lives. This inhibition occurs when we are ashamed, guilty, or afraid to express ourselves because we or our family might be judged by the disclosure. The rules of what is acceptable to share are covert and culturally determined. Disclosure depends upon cultural rules as well as idiosyncratic family rules.

Inhibition takes energy; it is a type of dysponesis (misdirected effort). Inhibition affects all parts of our physiology and functioning: from the blood vessels, the breathing pattern, and the immune system to the striate muscle system. When it involves the muscles, a person may brace and unknowingly tighten muscles such as those in the neck and shoulders. Holding back words and thoughts can easily become a pattern of holding (bracing) in the body. It takes effort to hold back, to distract ourselves, to not think or not feel. This causes both short-term biological changes and longer-term health consequences. Inhibition prevents us from truly understanding and assimilating the traumatic event. Talking or writing about a trauma offers the opportunity to reframe, to accept, to integrate, and to gain insight so that healing may occur. Sometimes just seeing, remembering, and experiencing the event from another perspective may evoke the wisdom we need to integrate and let go of the feelings and thoughts around the event. This is true whether the event is childhood sexual abuse, an earthquake, the loss of a spouse, or entering college.

James Pennebaker, a professor at Southern Methodist University in Dallas, Texas, has documented the health-promoting effects of "confession" (writing or talking about traumas) in a series of ingenious experiments. Typically, subjects were assigned to write (or talk into a tape recorder) for 20 minutes on 4 consecutive days. In one study subjects who were asked to disclose previously inhibited traumas showed pronounced improvement in immune function. The effects persisted for 6 weeks. College students who wrote about the trauma of coming to college decreased their health center visits by half in the 6 months following the experiment. (Subjects assigned to simply write about trivia showed no such changes.)

Given the opportunity to unburden, some subjects revealed a lot (high disclosers) while others did not (low disclosers). The high disclosers gained the largest health benefits. Those writing about traumas felt sad or depressed immediately afterward (and, for some, even throughout the whole 4-day period); these feelings soon gave way to feelings of increased well-being, however.

After disclosure, many people experience a sense of "freeing up." Most of us experience this when we come to a decision we have been wrestling with. During the period when we are mulling over the pros and cons, bodily discomfort, anxiety, and sleeplessness are common. Once we have made the decision, there is a sense of release—as if a burden has been lifted—even when we believe the choice made will result in discomfort.

Another interesting finding is that when people are actively inhibiting un-wanted thoughts and feelings, they tend to engage in activities requiring mindless or low-level thinking, such as housework, watching TV, eating, and strenuous exercise, rather than in activities requiring creative thinking or analytical problem solving. Pennebaker calls this "getting stupid and avoiding pain." Of course, drugs and alcohol may be used in the effort to numb pain and avoid thought, too. (Of all these strategies, physical exercise is undoubtedly the best alternative.) If there are unexpressed traumas and unwanted thoughts, you may have difficulty with high-level thinking. Perhaps this explains why 20% to 30% of the college students who wrote freely about traumas showed improvements (although slight) in their grades. In other studies subjects who had written about traumas showed increased congruence of brain waves between right and left hemispheres. Thus, writing seems to decrease the physiological work of inhibition and to increase our ability to understand, find meaning, manage situations, and complete unfinished business. It seems that by externalizing an event through writing or talking we gain a kind of distance from it, as if the expression allows a new reorganization of thought to occur.

Will Writing Benefit Your Ability to Cope?

People vary in the degree to which writing (or talking) about traumas will assist them. Consider writing if you can answer yes to any of the following questions:

- Do you have any issue you have never shared with another person, or have prevented yourself from thinking about, no matter how long ago it occurred?
- Do you have unwanted thoughts that crop up, including in your dreams?
- Are you still upset, grieving, or obsessed about a traumatic event a year and a half or more after it occurred?
- Are you currently undergoing a stressful situation or adjustment, such as being a college freshman or returning to college after years of being away?
- Do you sense you have "unfinished business"?
- Do you have trouble finding meaning in some traumatic event in your life?

A Few Cautions Before You Start

Writing is not a substitute for friends or a good therapist. Friends can provide emotional support and grounding in reality. If you are distraught, see a therapist. If you decide to talk to a confidant, be sure that your listener is nonjudgmental, that you can trust him or her to keep your secrets, that you are open and willing to listen to his or her confidences too and safeguard them, that you are not editing or distorting your expression to suit your audience, and that you are not doing this out of a desire to hurt your confidant. A therapist may be better suited for the listening role than many friends or family members.

Don't use writing as a substitute for action in situations over which you do have control. Don't write just to complain; that is counterproductive. Instead, express your deepest feelings and thoughts about the event. Beware of writing with intellectual detachment; try for self-reflectiveness. Notice feelings and ask yourself what makes you feel this way.

Instructions

1. Ideally, have a unique setting that is conducive to opening up. (People who rarely travel often open up to a complete stranger on an airplane, not only because they feel safely anonymous but because of the novelty of the situation.) Evening hours, dim lighting, candlelight, and complete privacy will all be helpful for letting go of inhibitions for your writing or tape-recording session. Set a specific time and location and keep it the same for each day's writing. Be sure there are no distracting sounds, smells, and sights.
2. Have complete privacy. Be sure that you KNOW you will not be seen, overheard, judged, or interrupted. For some people, anonymous public places such as a library are ideal locations; for others, sitting in the car with the doors locked offers a sense of security and privacy.
3. Decide whether you prefer to talk into a tape recorder or write and prepare by having a blank tape or plenty of paper and a pen available.
4. Set a timer for 20 minutes.
5. Once you begin, write or talk continuously for the whole 20 minutes about an upsetting or traumatic experience. Don't worry about grammar, spelling, or sentence structure. *Discuss your deepest thoughts and feelings about the experience.* You can write about anything you want but, whatever you choose, it should be something that has affected you very deeply. Ideally, it should be about something you have not discussed in detail with others. Let yourself go and touch the deepest emotions and thoughts you have. Write about what happened and how you felt about it, as well as how you feel about it now. You can write about different traumas during each session or the same one over the entire 4 days. If you run out of things to say, just keep going at the same pace and repeat what you have previously said or written. Write or speak it for *yourself*, not for anyone else or any

audience. This helps prevent you from editing it even subtly and rationalizing or justifying yourself to another person.

6. Don't be surprised if your writing style or voice on tape seems different from usual; this is normal.

7. Ask yourself the following questions while writing: What are my thoughts? How do they make me feel? Why do I feel this way?

8. If, for example, you choose to write about coming to college, you might consider addressing your thoughts and feelings about leaving your friends and parents, about adjusting to the various aspects of college, or even about your feelings of who you are or what you want to become.

9. Keep or destroy the written or audio material. Be sure if you keep the material that it is in a safe place and not left for others to discover and read or listen to.

10. Do not write for anyone but yourself. Do not turn in any of your writing or tapes. These are for you alone. However, *please be prepared to write about how you felt before and after the experience* for each day of your writing, along with any thoughts you have about the usefulness of the whole exercise. For that purpose, complete **Log Sheet: Freeing the Hidden Secrets: Practice 11**, in which you simply describe your emotional and mental states without revealing anything confidential. After one week, reflect upon your experience and complete **Worksheet: Integration: Practice 11.**

Optional: One month after completing the practice, describe how the practice changed your perspective on the experience. What other shifts in perspective took place? Although the instructions encourage either writing or talking about a hidden secret, there are numerous additional approaches to release and shift perspectives. Instead of writing or talking, express the experience in dance, photography, music, drawing, sculpture, sand painting, etc. In each case, be sure the focus is the expression of something that has affected you deeply. This nonverbal expression involves the intuitive and creative component that is within each of us. It is in connecting with this intuitive/creative force that healing occurs.

Name _____ Date _____

Log Sheet   Freeing the Hidden Secrets: Practice 11

For each of the 4 days you write, describe how you felt before and after the experience. (Reminder: you are *not* being asked to disclose any of the contents of your private writing.)

Day 1   Before: _____

Date _____   _____

_____

_____

_____

After: _____

_____

_____

_____

_____

_____

_____

Day 2   Before: _____

Date _____   _____

_____

_____

_____

After: _____

_____

_____

_____

_____

_____

_____

Day 3   Before: _____

Date _____   _____

_____

_____

_____

After: _____

_____

_____

_____

_____

_____

Day 4   Before: _____

Date _____   _____

_____

_____

_____

After: _____

_____

_____

_____

_____

_____

Comments: _____

_____

_____

_____

_____

_____

_____

_____

Worksheet   Integration: Freeing the Hidden Secrets: Practice 11

One week after completing the writing exercise, describe how the writing changed your perspective on the experience you wrote about. What other shifts in perspective took place?

_____

_____

_____

_____

_____

_____

_____

_____

_____

_____

_____

_____

_____

_____

_____

_____

_____

_____

_____

_____

_____

_____

_____

_____

_____

_____

_____

_____

_____

CONVERTING THE ADVANTAGES OF ILLNESS: PRACTICE 12

Now when my eye fuzzes up, I know that it is telling me to slow down, stop judging people and not be so hard on myself.
Client with Multiple Sclerosis

My heart attack made me ask myself was my work worth dying for. It made me realize how estranged I had become from my children. Looking back, it gave me a second chance with life and my family.
Client with Heart Disease

Each of us would like to be well and healthy; however, health-promoting practices may at times be more difficult, demanding, and/or painful than continuing our present illness-producing or maintaining patterns. When we look back at a past illness, we can often see that the illness brought with it certain benefits and/or advantages. For example, being sick may have allowed us to excuse ourselves from work or family obligations and to experience love and care. Being ill may allow time for reflection or breaks from boring routines. A major or life-threatening illness may force us to make changes in relationships, work, and life direction. After all, if our survival is at stake, why put up with what is killing us?

It is interesting to consider that our bodies may be wiser than we are and that when we get off track—for example, by making the wrong decision, by overworking, or by staying in a dead-end job or abusive relationship—our bodies let us know and demand that we stop doing whatever it is. Have you ever wondered why if your job demands a lot of speaking or telephone work, you seem to get laryngitis (rather than, say, a broken ankle)? Rather than getting angry at our "uncooperative" body parts, we might ask them, "How do I need to take care of you better?" or even "How are you taking care of me?" To quote Norman Cousins: "When we have a health disorder, we should ask what our bodies are doing right to adapt to a situation, and not what is wrong with our bodies." By identifying the advantages of illness, we may be able to change our behavior, learn from the illness experience, and mobilize our innate healing potential.

Sometimes we develop illness as a conditioned response to certain events or stressful situations. One theory of allergic reactivity is that when a young, sensitive, and vulnerable child is subjected to a traumatic event, such as parental fighting, his or her body reacts dramatically. The child's immune system goes on the alert to find the antigen that might be responsible for the reaction but finds, say, only cat dandruff in the child's sinuses. The immune system mounts an all-out attack on this antigen, leading to sneezing, wheezing, and so forth. If this combination of events happens a few times, the immune response becomes conditioned and will activate whenever cat hair is around—and/or whenever emotional stress occurs. In addition, if the child's allergic response leads to the parents dropping their argument and uniting to care for him or her, the response is further reinforced. When such children grow up, this allergic response is no longer so useful in getting their (or their family's) needs met, so it may disappear naturally. Or the allergy may "outlive its usefulness" and disappear when the adult understands its origin.

We live in a culture that places little importance on inner development and, indeed, tells us there is too much else to do to take any time for it. Regular time set aside for reflection and expression—for example, journal writing or an emotional support group or creative artistic expression—is not a part of most people's lives. Yet this type of inner work may well be vital to our health, both emotional and physical. When we stray too far from the path of the heart, getting caught up in a rat race of "have to's" and "shoulds," we get sick. And there are many wonderful stories of people healing—even from usually fatal illnesses—when they rediscover and begin to pursue what is truly meaningful to them. This has been graphically described by Evy MacDonald in her lectures and public appearances. She is a remarkable nurse administrator who completely recovered from amyotrophic lateral sclerosis (ALS). After receiving the gloomy prognosis for this usually fatal disease, she decided that before she died she wanted to learn to love herself unconditionally. Previously, she had always been too focused on outward achievement to be aware of her inner pain; having a life-threatening illness enabled her to turn her life around. She views the illness as a gift that enabled her to heal her self-hatred and transform her life.

Evy MacDonald emphasizes that each person's path of healing is unique. From our perspective, illness is complex and multicausal. In almost all cases, it is the interaction of genetics, environment, psychosocial variables, and the like. Even when we take responsibility to mobilize our self-healing, it may *not* result in improved health. It may, however, help us to grow.

The purpose of this exercise is to explore the advantages and benefits associated with some past or possibly present illness and to develop a strategy by which we can experience the benefits associated with the disease process without having the disease. For example, if an illness allowed me time to be by myself or to read or to watch TV without feeling guilty, how can I now develop a strategy that would include some "time out"—a time period in which I could take care of those needs?

Begin by identifying the advantages of illness and then develop a strategy by which you may experience these advantages without being sick; use the worksheet entitled **Converting the Advantages of Illness: Practice 12.** Each time you create the benefits, complete **Log Sheet: Practice 12.** At the end of the week review your experience and answer the **Questions: Practice 12.** Then meet with your group and complete **Discussion and Conclusions: Practice 12.**

Optional: After having completed Chapter 3 of this workbook, review your experiences. Write about them as suggested in the section "Reflection and Integration: Summarizing Your Experiences" in Chapter 1. This process allows an opportunity to reflect and integrate your experience.

Name _____ Date _____

Worksheet Converting the Advantages of Illness: Practice 12

1. Describe some past or present illness or injury: _____
   _____
   _____
   _____

2. List the advantages or benefits gained when you were ill or injured:
   A. _____
   _____
   _____
   _____
   _____

   B. _____
   _____
   _____
   _____
   _____

   C. _____
   _____
   _____
   _____

3. Select one of the advantages you gained when you were ill and develop a
   strategy by which you can continue to experience that benefit. (For example:
   An advantage of being ill was having my mother cook for me. My mother
   lives a long way away, so it's not practical to go home for a meal. Instead, I
   can either ask my best friend to cook for me or take myself out for dinner. I
   don't have to get sick in order to enjoy the dinner; in fact, I might enjoy it more
   if I'm NOT sick!) Describe the advantage you picked and how you are going
   to implement the strategy to gain that advantage during the week. Be sure
   you include how, when, where, and with whom:

_____
_____
_____
_____
_____
_____

4. How might you try to talk yourself out of doing the exercise during the week and how will you counter your own self-talk?

_____
_____
_____
_____
_____
_____

5. Now share and role-play your strategy with the members in your group and ask them to play devil's advocate. The role of your group members is to help you finalize your procedure and discover possible ways by which you may fail to implement your strategy. With their help, describe the restructured procedure you will practice during the week.

_____
_____
_____
_____
_____
_____
_____
_____
_____
_____
_____
_____
_____

Name _____ Date _____

Log Sheet   Converting the Advantages of Illness: Practice 12

Describe when, where, and what you experienced when you practiced your advantages-of-illness exercise. (For some, this exercise needs to be done only once or twice.)

Date _____

_____
_____
_____
_____
_____
_____
_____
_____
_____
_____
_____
_____
_____
_____

Date _____

_____
_____
_____
_____
_____
_____
_____
_____
_____
_____
_____
_____
_____
_____

Date _____

Date _____

Date _____

Name _____ Date _____

Questions   Converting the Advantages of Illness: Practice 12

1. How was it for you to receive the benefits of illness without having to be sick?

_____

_____

_____

_____

_____

_____

2. What insights from this exercise might you incorporate into your life in order to reduce the "need" for illness?

_____

_____

_____

_____

_____

_____

3. What problems/challenges occurred and how did you cope with them?

_____

_____

_____

_____

_____

4. How would you have done this exercise differently?

_____

_____

_____

_____

_____

Discussion and Conclusions   Converting the Advantages of
Illness: Practice 12

1. What benefits did the group members notice as a result of the practice?

_____

_____

_____

_____

_____

_____

2. Describe common themes in the strategies that the group members adopted
   to achieve the advantages of illness without being sick.

_____

_____

_____

_____

_____

_____

3. Among group members, how were the experiences of this week's practice
   related to past and/or present illness patterns and beliefs about responsibility
   and/or control over health?

_____

_____

_____

_____

_____

_____

4. Topics for which instructor consultation would be helpful:

_____

_____

List your group members: _____ _____

_____ _____ _____

_____ _____ _____

SUGGESTED READINGS

Beck, A. T., Rush, A. J., Shaw, B. F., & Emery, G. (1979). *Cognitive Therapy of Depression.* New York: Guilford.
Borysenko, J. (1987). *Minding the Body, Mending the Mind.* Reading, MA: Addison-Wesley.
Burns, D. (1980). *Feeling Good: The New Mood Therapy.* New York: Signet.
Davis, M., Eshelman, E. R., & McKay, M. (1982). *The Relaxation and Stress Reduction Workbook.* Oakland, CA: New Harbinger.
Dobson, K. S. (Ed.). (1988). *Handbook of Cognitive–Behavioral Therapies.* New York: Guilford.
Easwaran, E. (1981). *Dialogue with Death.* Petaluma, CA: Nilgiri Press.
Kabat-Zinn, J. (1990). *Full Catastrophe Living.* New York: Delacorte Press.
Lynch, J. J. (1985). *The Language of the Heart.* New York: Basic Books.
Pennebaker, J. W. (1991). *Opening Up: The Healing Power of Confiding in Others.* New York: Morrow.
Seligman, M. E. P. (1991). *Learned Optimism.* New York: Knopf.
Smith, M. J. (1975). *When I Say No, I Feel Guilty.* New York: Bantam Books.
Tannen, D. (1990). *You Just Don't Understand.* New York: Morrow.

Chapter 4
Self-Healing Through Imagery and Behavior Change

Movement in the depth of being is the manner in which the psyche performs its directive role in man. The content of this movement is imagery.

IRA PROGOFF

Imagination is a good horse to carry you over the ground, not a magic carpet to take you away from the world of possibilities.

ROBERTSON DAVIES

MOBILIZING HEALING WITH IMAGERY AND BEHAVIOR CHANGE

I am part of the world—the universe. I am connected to the yellow healing energies and the blue peaceful calm. All flow through me and around me. I am whole. I am good. I am part of the world. The dark clouds are also part of the world—they will be there but only along with the blue and yellow.

I see myself as a seed. The roots have been growing for a long time but I feel like I've just cracked the seedpod and am reaching for the light. The drought, the rain, the wind, the calm—all are parts of life that affect the seed—all help it to become stronger in some way. These things are not so much to be feared—as to be understood.

JANICE METTLER

We believe that all of us can mobilize our self-healing potential, although this does not mean that we will get physically healthier. In fact, we will all die. Nor is it possible to resolve all psychological and social conflicts or problems. However, we are all capable of moving toward wholeness and integration.

In beginning the self-healing process, there are two important components: imagery and behavior change. Imagery is very important because of its potential for bringing insights from the unconscious mind into awareness. Whenever illness or other forms of imbalance are present, we could go to someone outside ourselves, such as a doctor or therapist, to get a diagnosis and a prescription for how to get well; or we could choose to tap into that part of ourselves that truly understands what the problem is and how to resolve it. Insights gained through imagery exploration may then direct us to make certain behavior changes involving rest, diet, exercise, work/career, relationships, and so on. Sometimes there are surprises, sometimes not. Often the insights that come from imagery sessions help provide the truly inner-directed motivation to make the necessary lifestyle changes.

What Is Imagery?

Imagery is the direct language of the unconscious and the autonomic nervous system. Although most people associate imagery with the visual domain, we use the term in a broader sense. Images can be visual, olfactory, tactile, kinesthetic, or auditory. They may be directly descriptive or allegorical. Imagery can be passively observed or overtly acted out, guided or spontaneous. Imagery represents the symbolic communication of body/mind/spirit. It is our belief that through imagery we can access the deepest levels of our self-knowledge and awareness. Bodily symptoms can be thought of as communications from the unconscious. "Decoding" these symptoms into messages we can understand can occur through imagery.

When we use the term *imagery* in this workbook, it usually means spontaneous as opposed to a guided or preconceived visualization. Visualizations are images that are consciously created and directed; they can be very helpful. The exercises in this section emphasize tapping creative and healing potentials by means of unedited spontaneity in the imagery. Often, visualization and imagery may be combined. For example, a guided visualization may suggest that you are about to meet a wise being, without telling you anything descriptive about this being, such as gender, age, or even whether this being is an animal or a human. All the specifics are allowed to arise spontaneously in your mind.

The right and left hemispheres of the brain seem to have somewhat specialized functions. While the left hemisphere is responsible for speech, analysis, and logic, the right hemisphere is involved with images, emotions, the larger picture, and relationships between events and between people. In our society we tend to value the rational linear, logical thought of the left hemisphere; therefore, we are usually not in touch with the insight and wisdom that the right hemisphere can provide. However, when we become deeply relaxed in body and mind, the censorship of the left hemisphere loosens and we can access insight and wisdom from the right hemisphere by tuning into images. "Imagery lets you communicate with your own silent mind in its native tongue" (Rossman, 1987, p. 25). Ideally, in this simplified model the right and left hemispheres work as a team. The right gives guidance and the left creates the will, intention, and real-world behavior changes.

Imagery is used to become aware of the underlying meaning of illnesses or as a tool to enhance the healing process. Imagery, like dreams, offers insight into patterns underlying the messages of the body. In addition, it is one of the approaches by which people can actively, and in a self-accepting way, participate in their own reintegration. Moreover, in the act of imaging you may rehearse and make easier a new behavior. Benefits usually accrue if the imaging is practiced often and with an openness to new insights. It is used in a wide array of areas— from psychotherapy, personal goal setting, and self-healing to enhancing peak performance (athletes often call this type of practice "visual motor behavior rehearsal").

Imagery, combined with acting on our goals, gives us the experience and confidence that change is possible. In the act of doing, we *know*—not just believe— that we can grow and change. Athletic, theater, and musical performers mentally rehearse exactly how they will act. They create in their minds visual, kinesthetic, auditory, and olfactory sensations as they imagine themselves performing perfectly. As they mentally rehearse, their bodies react as if the performance is actually occurring. The actual performance is the next step.

Imagery is usually practiced after relaxation has been mastered. For many people, a regular relaxation practice is all that is needed to relieve or prevent the majority of symptoms; for others, relaxation sets the stage for a deeper exploration of problem areas through imagery. The healing can include reduction of physical symptoms, accepting who and what you are, transforming negative mental and emotional patterns, or integrating new behavior patterns such as increasing exercise or improving diet to enhance health.

If you have led a sedentary life and have no particular illness problems, you may simply feel that your life would be healthier if you exercised. Exercise, then, can be your self-healing practice. Mental rehearsal of yourself exercising and enjoying it can be a motivator. Some people include imagery as a complement to their medical treatment, such as chemotherapy for cancer. Many have reported that by taking care of one symptomatic area in a holistic way they improved their general health and well-being. When we begin to trust and follow our inner promptings (intuition), rather than acting from "shoulds" and expectations, we encourage healing. How do we know whether to trust an impulse? Is it intuition or conditioning/habits/desires? Follow those "gut" feelings and look at the results! If the results enhance your wholeness, that is good evidence that you followed your intuition.

The self-healing process is based upon a sequence of steps. These steps will first be listed and then described in detail.

1. *Imagery Exploration: Answers from the Unconscious.* For one week allow spontaneous images to come each day. Either ask the question "What do I need to know or do for my own self-healing?" or hold conversations with an inner guide (see sections **Exploration Script** and **Inner Guide Script** in this chapter).

2. *Developing a Self-Healing Strategy.* On the basis of information you discover during imagery exploration,[1] include some or all of the following steps:
   a. Reviewing the insights from imagery
   b. Reading up on the area of concern
   c. Setting goals and priorities
   d. Monitoring baseline data
   e. Arranging new behavioral cues
   f. Planning reinforcers
   g. Planning ahead for relapses
3. *Imagery for Self-Healing.* Begin with the image of illness and develop a process for healing that is ongoing and prevents relapses. Finally, imagine yourself integrated and whole.
4. *Carrying Out and Adapting Your Strategy.* Using self-devised log forms, maintain an ongoing evaluation of your success or failure in achieving your goals; modify your strategy when necessary.
5. *Integrating Your Experience.* Summarize what you have learned.

IMAGERY EXPLORATION: ANSWERS FROM THE UNCONSCIOUS: PRACTICE 13

Imagery exploration is based on the observation that our unconscious can communicate and be accessed through imagery or dreams. This communication may be more accessible when we are quiet (centered) and not distracted by external cues or internal emotions and desires. Imagery is then a communication from our intuitive and creative self. At times, symptoms and problems are messages that prod us to make changes in our lives.

Do not have an agenda or try to construct images. Be open to novelty and surprise. Remember, images need not be visual. They may be kinesthetic or auditory sensations or a felt sense. Don't judge your experience. If your attention wanders, bring it gently back to the question. Even fleeting images or feelings may be important, so record them faithfully. Some things that are puzzling to you now may later make sense. You can explore the previous day's images by asking open-ended questions about them during the practice. It may be useful to ask, "When did this problem develop? Why do I have it?"

Many healing traditions call upon a wise inner guide or advisor. This being—in the form of a friendly animal, a guardian angel, a religious figure, a wise old man or woman, a radiant light, or simply a voice (the form does not matter)—is compassionate and loving and understands everything about your problem or symptom and how to heal it. This wise being is actually a part of you: the part that truly knows how you can assist in your own healing. You may also have more than one guide. Accept whatever image comes to you. The insight or images you access may direct you to something other than what you would have chosen for your self-healing project. For instance, a woman who thought that her self-healing would involve dieting to lose weight discovered through her imagery that the most important thing was learning new ways to nurture the child within her and treat herself well. These new ways did not involve food but included long, hot bubble baths, drawing, and going to the beach.

Accept the spontaneous images. They are meaningful although they may sometimes appear to come from left field. For example, one woman wanted to use imagery to enlarge her breasts. The image that came up—large, droopy breasts like her mother's—surprised her. She felt disgusted by the image. As a small child, she might have thought: "I do not want droopy breasts when I am my mother's age. Therefore, my breasts will stay small and not grow large!" For her, self-healing was accepting the images of her own and her mother's body.

Another woman observed that each time she explored ways to reduce her sugar intake, an image of her ex-lover appeared:

> My relationship with this man and our consequent separation involved a lot of emotional turbulence, and I soon realized that although our connection ran very deep, on one level he was a means of filling a void within myself, like sugar was. Furthermore, I would often find myself stuffing my face with sweets whenever I was feeling hurt over this relationship. This realization helped me to gain an increased awareness of my thoughts and feelings surrounding my sugar habit. . . .The objects of our addictions take many forms, but they all seem to be a means of connection to something we don't find in our lives. I have begun to probe more deeply into the spiritual question that is the human condition: How can we find love, how can we feel connected? . . . Meditation has helped me to address this question by awakening an awareness in me that enables me to go into each experience fully, to be completely present in the moment, and to observe how I am feeling in the moment . . . I feel that as I bring more awareness to my life through the integration of mind/body and spirituality, my compulsive behaviors, including my sugar addiction, will eventually disappear.

Instructions

Each day begin with your favorite relaxation practice, which you synthesized during Practice 8, or use the printed relaxation script. After you have relaxed and feel peaceful, continue either with the **Exploration Script,** which consists of a series of open-ended questions, or with the **Inner Guide Script** (both are presented in the next section of this chapter). You may want to adapt the questions in the exploration script to the area you have selected for healing. These two sample scripts were adapted from a very helpful book, *Healing Yourself,* by Martin Rossman (1987). Allow images to arise spontaneously for 10 to 15 minutes. In some cases nothing comes up. That is equally OK. Just continue with the practice. We suggest you try out each of these imagery explorations at least once and go with the one you find most helpful. After each practice draw, sketch, or in some other way express the images. At the end of this week's practice integrate the observations and develop your self-healing project.

If an uncomfortable, unfriendly, or critical figure arises with the inner guide imagery, ask it to go away and request another guide. (For further suggestions, see Rossman's *Healing Yourself.*) If you choose to draw or paint your image, be sure to have your materials available before starting your relaxation.

Express the Images

Each day after you have gone through the script, find a way to express the important images. You can draw or sketch them in color, compose a musical composition, act them out in dance, and so forth. Remember, not everyone receives visual images. If your information came as words, sounds, or feelings, these are fine. Describe them briefly in your log notes.

If you do draw or paint, you might consider using your nondominant hand, which is in closest communication with the nondominant (right) hemisphere of the brain. This technique has been taught by Lucia Capacchione and is beautifully described and illustrated in *Recovery of Your Inner Child* and *The Power of Your Other Hand*. You might also write next to your drawing a few words that seem appropriate, while still using your nondominant hand. Be sure not to judge these drawings or writings as clumsy or childish. These are powerful ways to enhance the imagery experience. To clarify the insight gained from imagery, write a single sentence that most clearly expresses that insight.

When beginning to pay more attention to spontaneous imagery, many people report that their nighttime dreaming becomes more vivid and meaningful and that they remember their dreams more easily. This may be because through imagery explorations we are encouraging and increasing our access to previously unconscious material.

Answers from the Unconscious: Scripts

Have drawing or painting materials ready. Get comfortable in a sitting position, and let your body relax and rest. Allow your eyes to close. For the next few minutes, recreate the sensations you experienced in your previous relaxation practices.

Insert your Personal Relaxation Script (from Practice 8) or continue with the following relaxation script.

> Relax all over; allow a pleasant heaviness to develop . . . Take a couple of deep, full breaths and feel yourself letting go with each exhalation . . . Allow the comfortable sensations of warmth to flow through your entire body . . . Let go of any unnecessary tension and take the time to attend to each part of your body . . . Invite your feet and legs to relax, gently noting any areas where there is tension and just releasing it . . . Allow your thighs and buttocks to relax, then your pelvis and lower back . . . Feel your abdomen expand with your slow, easy breaths . . . Let go of tension, being aware of any area of your body where there is a need for healing. . . Relaxing the organs within your abdomen and chest . . . Relax your back . . . Feel more and more comfortably relaxed, letting go of your shoulders and neck, relaxing your arms and hands . . . Feel the warm relaxation flowing, allowing your forehead and eye muscles to let go, your jaws,

throat, and face to relax . . . Feel your breath flowing easily in and out.

And now find yourself in a special inner place of relaxation and healing, a place where you feel calm, safe, and secure . . . Notice what your senses are taking in: colors, sights, sounds, textures, aromas . . . Breathe in the peacefulness, the quiet, soothing atmosphere of this place, and find a spot in which to settle down, where you feel centered and comfortable . . . You might say to yourself: "I am now deeply relaxed in a calm, peaceful state of mind. My body feels comfortable and quiet. My mind is clear and open to images that will be helpful to me."

Continue with either the Exploration Script or Inner Guide Script.

Exploration Script.   When you feel ready, bring your awareness to your own area of concern, the symptom or problem that you would like to heal . . . While you remain comfortably relaxed, allow any image to emerge that represents this symptom or problem and accept whatever image comes, whether it is symbolic or realistic, familiar or strange . . . Observe, feel, touch it from different perspectives and note how large it is, what shape and color it has, and whether it moves or not . . . Notice where the problem seems to be, how and where you feel it inside yourself . . . Does it have a sound or vibration? . . . A smell or a taste?

And now ask, "What do I need to know or do for my own self-healing?" And let another image arise that represents the process of healing . . . Allow this image of healing to become vivid and bright and clear . . . See it, feel it, and experience it. . . What part do you need to play in this healing process? . . . Observe this process for as long as you like and then slowly and gently begin to feel yourself as you rest on the chair . . . Become aware of the your toes and wiggle them; gently move your fingers . . . Give yourself a slow, comfortable stretch. . . Breathe fully and open your eyes when you feel ready.

Inner Guide Script.   As you relax and rest in your peaceful place of healing, you now become aware of another being who is approaching, yet waiting to be invited to join you . . . It could be a person, an animal, a light . . . Just accept whatever image comes, as long as it feels safe for you . . . As this being comes nearer, you notice that it appears to be kind and gentle and wise . . . This guide knows you very well . . . And so, if it feels right to you, invite this being to be with you awhile in your special place . . . Take a moment to study your guide, noticing everything about it . . . Feel the loving presence . . . And now, with your area of concern in mind, ask your guide any question that comes up . . . You might want to ask why you have this problem or what steps you can take to assist your own healing . . . And wait for an answer to come . . . Allow it to communicate with you in whatever way seems natural, which may not be in words . . . Answers may also come at a later time, such as in a dream or while relaxing later . . . You may ask any other question you wish, to gain more clarity . . . And again, be open to the answer in whatever form it may come . . . If you receive advice you feel hesitant to follow, know that you can ask for further explanation, either now or later, and that you can ask for reassurance that the advice will be helpful.

And now thank your guide and say good-bye, knowing that you can make contact again at any time when you are relaxed . . . Watch as your guide leaves and once again feel the beautiful serenity of your special place enfolding you . . . Breathe easily and become more aware of your body . . . Slowly wiggle your fingers and toes, breathing deeply . . . Open your eyes when you are ready.

Each day right after your imagery exercise (and drawing), complete **Log Sheet: Practice 13.** At the end of the week answer **Questions: Practice 13.** Meet with your group and complete **Discussion and Conclusions: Practice 13.**

Name _____ Date _____

Log Sheet Answers from the Unconscious: Practice 13

After each daily practice session (a) describe your questions from the exploration or dialogue with the internal guide, (b) describe your imagery, and (c) write the sentence that most clearly describes the insight gained from the imagery.

Day 1   a. _____

Date _____   _____

    b. _____

_____

_____

    c. _____

_____

Day 2   a. _____

Date _____   _____

    b. _____

_____

_____

    c. _____

_____

Day 3   a. _____

Date _____   _____

    b. _____

_____

_____

    c. _____

_____

Day 4   a. _____

Date _____   _____

    b. _____

169

_____

_____

     c. _____

_____

Day 5   a. _____

Date _____   _____

     b. _____

_____

_____

     c. _____

_____

Day 6   a. _____

Date _____   _____

     b. _____

_____

_____

     c. _____

_____

_____

Day 7   a. _____

Date _____   _____

     b. _____

_____

_____

     c. _____

_____

Name _____ Date _____

Questions   Answers from the Unconscious: Practice 13

1. What benefits occurred as a result of your practice?

_____

_____

_____

2. What were the common themes of your imagery?

_____

_____

_____

3. How did the two approaches (exploration and inner guide) affect you?

_____

_____

_____

4. What were the common themes in the sentences that you wrote in your log sheets?

_____

_____

_____

5. What did you learn from drawing? Did you use your nondominant hand? What other forms of expression did you use?

_____

_____

_____

6. What problems/challenges occurred and how did you solve them?

_____

_____

_____

Name_____ Date_____

Discussion and Conclusions Answers from the Unconscious:
Practice 13

1. What benefits did the group members notice as a result of the practice?

_____

_____

_____

_____

2. How did the images offer insight into the explored questions and problems?
Share drawings and other productions with others in the group for feedback.

_____

_____

_____

_____

3. Among group members, how easy or difficult was it to allow and capture
spontaneous images? How helpful was the conversation with an inner guide?

_____

_____

_____

_____

4. How did writing a single sentence after each practice help develop insight?

_____

_____

_____

5. Topics for which instructor consultation would be helpful:

_____

_____

List your group members: _____ _____

_____ _____ _____

_____ _____ _____

DEVELOPING A SELF-HEALING STRATEGY

Scientific discovery is 1% inspiration and 99% perspiration.

This next phase involves transforming insight from your imagery exploration into an action plan. Having insight is fun and inspiring, but it is through action that we truly transform ourselves. If we do not act upon insights, we tend to disconnect from our inner knowing. Taking charge and developing a self-healing strategy means that you are becoming the master of your own ship. No longer are you adrift, pushed around, and buffeted by myriad thoughts and stimuli. The aim of this section is to develop an action plan and begin the self-healing practice. Read the background material carefully and then develop your plan. Many of these concepts have been derived from an outstanding text by Watson and Tharp (1981), *Self-Directed Behavior: Self-Modification for Personal Adjustment*. We recommend that you look at this text if you would like additional information.

Review the Insights from Imagery

Go over your responses from the previous section and list a few ways by which you might translate these insights into practical action. Brainstorm by writing down as many ways as you can think of to put your plan into action. You might want to do this with your small group or a friend. Brainstorming means that even the wildest ideas are allowed and written down, with the aim of generating many possibilities in a short time. Then, look over your options. Which would be the simplest, easiest, most practical, most fun? Choose one or two.

Read Up on the Area of Concern[2]

Become informed about the problem to which you plan to apply your self-healing practices. For example, if your imagery guided you to work with your sore back, research both standard, or allopathic, medical approaches (e.g., orthopedics and physical therapy) and complementary, or alternative, approaches (e.g., chiropractic, Feldenkrais, or massage). By exploring and investigating appropriate treatment approaches, you can begin to make informed choices. You can question your allopathic or alternative health care provider on the risks and benefits of any proposed strategy. You will then be in a good position to devise your self-healing strategy, which may or may not use allopathic approaches.

Set Goals and Priorities

If you want your dream to be
Build it slow and surely
Small beginning, greater end
Heartfelt work grows purely.
        "Stone by Stone" by Donovan,
from the film *Brother Sun, Sister Moon*

Set realistic and, if possible, quantifiable goals. Define your goals clearly, in terms of particular behaviors in particular situations. That will make your progress much easier to measure. After all, being able to see measurable evidence of change, even if it is small, is a wonderful incentive to help keep you going in a new (and perhaps less comfortable) behavior. If, for example, you would like to be more outgoing, you'll first want to decide what outgoing behavior means to you. Perhaps it means smiling and making eye contact with an increasing number of people each day or speaking up in class more times each week or starting more conversations with people at work.

It's easier to increase desirable behavior than to decrease undesirable behavior. For example, if you'd like to stop biting your nails, increase the number of times you engage in different behaviors with your hands, such as using an emery board or giving yourself a brief hand massage. If the desired behavior is incompatible with the problem behavior, so much the better. Saying something pleasant to yourself or another person is incompatible with saying something critical.

Set your goal on behaviors that you can monitor and control. For example, if your goal is to lose weight, break that down into several subgoals that are expressed as specific behaviors in particular situations, for example, getting up from the table and going for a walk instead of staying for dessert, relaxing and acknowledging emotions when anxious or upset, beginning an exercise program, or substituting more vegetables for high-fat foods. If you get stuck on what your subgoals need to be, try brainstorming, that is, scribbling down any and all ideas, no matter how wild or impractical, and selecting later.

If your goal is to remove a wart from a finger using imagery, your behavioral subgoals might include daily relaxation and visualization of the wart shrinking. You could also count every time during the day you remember the thought and image of the wart dissolving and your finger being smooth and totally healthy. You may want to monitor thoughts that are self-defeating and those that are supportive of healing.

Remember to start with small, easy to achieve goals; then move on to more challenging ones. Start with the behavior change that is the most fun, easiest, and most appealing; the others will follow more readily when you have already gotten yourself moving. For example, exercise leads to a better self-image and body, which then makes it easier not to eat compulsively.

Collect Baseline Data

Before beginning the self-healing project, establish a baseline of where you are now. Whatever behavior or other data your decide to monitor, attempt to be as specific as possible. Ask when, where, what, and with whom the behavior occurs; what precedes it; and how it changes your or others' behavior afterward. For example, if you have a migraine headache twice a week, record the time and place of occurrence along with all the other situational and behavioral information you can come up with. For example, your notes might read as follows: "Finished a 10-page paper, what a relief, after 4 days of intense effort. Migraine, pain about 8 on a scale of 1 to 10. Began the night after I turned in the paper and lasted until the next day at 1:00 P.M., family tiptoed around and didn't disturb me."

In order to establish a baseline and later monitor progress, you may want to devise your own log format. For example, one woman who was monitoring negative self-talk carried a small notepad around with her at all times and jotted down each negative thought; then she immediately rephrased it in a more positive and rational way. She also used the notepad to record affirmations and looked at them a few times each day. One person devised a food diary with spaces for recording his emotions and thoughts about the food, as well as how hungry he was, the time, and so forth.

These measures can be divided into objective and subjective categories. Objective measures tend to be quantifiable and include such variables as weight, number of laps run in 10 minutes, blood pressure level, and so on. Subjective measures tend to be ratings and description of feelings, such as intensity of depression, alertness, or pain.

Here are a few more examples of baseline and continuing measurement strategies that others have used:

- Simple tally sheet of marks to register each time a problem behavior occurs per day, with a graph at the end of the week
- A mood-rating chart (used by a woman working on overcoming depression)
- Inkprints of a wart on a fingertip, showing its shrinkage each week
- A series of pictures of body image, beginning with a whale and ending with a small fish (see the last section of this chapter, "Integrating Your Experience")
- Measurements of range of motion in an area of the back that did not move normally
- Self-rating scales for pain intensity (important to rate and record because when you're not in pain, it's hard to remember how it felt when you were, and vice versa)
- Testimonials from friend, roommate, or spouse offering another's view of changes observed in you (see "Integrating Your Experience"). If your behavior is quite automatic or unconscious, you may want to enlist the help of others to point out when you do it (gently and tactfully, of course, not punitively!).

During the period in which you record your baseline data, which is typically a week or two, you are just observing. However, the mere act of recording may also change the behavior in the desired direction by bringing more awareness into it and thus making it less automatic. Remember that statements you make to yourself are also a form of behavior. You may be monitoring a symptom to begin with; in addition, you may decide to observe your own behavior and/or inner language that precedes or in some way seems to support the symptom. (See Sample Daily Log, by a student with multiple subgoals.)

Sample Daily Log

Date: _Thurs., Nov. 24_

Diet: Water (glasses) _2_

Salty foods _yes_

Wine _Champagne III   wine III_

Caffeine _coffee   HHH I   Coke III_

Fats _yes_

Exercise: Type _dance_

How long? _20 minutes_

Heart rates _____

Time of day _____

Relaxation: Type _____ _none_

Time of day _____

How long? _____

How effective? _____

Sleep: Bedtime _2 AM_

Wake time _8 AM_

Hours _6_

Quality _ok_

Other: Any symptoms? _still PMS_

If so, what and when? _____

Idea of nature of symptom _____

General
well-being: Moods _moody_

Physical _very tired_

Spiritual _down_

Comments
on today: _dress rehearsal   11/3   20 people to dinner   busy day   ate far too much_

If your goal is to stop smoking, collect data first. Discover how many cigarettes you smoke a day and in which situations you want the cigarette most (with coffee, with alcohol, with certain friends, when others light up, or when you're bored, tense, angry, etc.). In other words, what are your triggers or cues?

If your goal is to control your temper, ask yourself, "Is there a chain of events that leads inevitably to the problem behavior?" For example: "I come home from work tired and cranky, the kids are whining or fighting, I start hurrying to fix dinner without taking a break, I feel hassled and pressured, and then I yell at one of the kids. If I interrupt this chain by taking even a few minutes to relax before I jump into fixing dinner, there is less likelihood that I'll lose my temper. If I can even catch myself feeling pressured and substitute another thought, I can break the chain." Observations such as these will provide valuable information to help you devise a strategy for success.

If it is some form of compulsive behavior—such as overeating, alcohol use, smoking, or drug use—that you are seeking to decrease or eliminate, be aware that the behavior is probably taking place in order to suppress some unpleasant or unacceptable feelings you are having. By keeping good records of the thoughts and feelings that typically precede this behavior, you can discover their nature; then ask yourself how you might accept yourself for having those feelings and take care of yourself in a better way. Get emotional support; avoid guilt. A student observed, "Obsessions are ways to remove yourself from yourself because you're not comfortable with who you are and what you're feeling." Acknowledge your feelings; nourish yourself emotionally.

In this self-observation period, also make note of the consequences of your problem behavior or symptom. Honestly list the advantages and disadvantages (see "Converting the Advantages of Illness: Practice 12"). Spelling out the consequences may help you increase your motivation for change and may uncover the factors that undermine change. For example, does smoking given you a chance for time out and reflection? This is a reinforcer that helps maintain the smoking habit. Is there another way you can give yourself this time out?

Arrange New Behavioral Cues

Arrange new cues to help create the positive behavior. Once you are aware of the situations and cues that lead to the unwanted behaviors, you can start rearranging them. You can substitute positive self-talk for negative. Ask yourself, "Is my self-talk making my desired behavior more—or less—likely? Is my inner language rewarding or punishing my behavior?" If you're saying, "She won't like me," stop it and say, "I know what to do. Relax, smile, make eye contact, say hello." This is called self-instruction. Choose situations that will support, not undermine, the new behavior you are cultivating (e.g., a new ex-smoker can choose to be around nonsmokers, and can choose to avoid puffing friends, alcohol, and parties, if those were previously identified as important cues or triggers for the desire to smoke).

You can pause and do a QR (see "Quick and Warm: Practice 6") when you encounter one of your cues. This is especially important if your problem involves anxiety or tension. Think, "What other alternative do I have besides getting into an argument (or taking a drink or reaching for a cigarette)?" Or you might think, "I choose to focus on what I like about this person instead of getting into an argument" or "I choose to drink a glass of sparkling soda water instead of a beer (or chew a piece of gum instead of smoking a cigarette)." Thus, you are interrupting an automatic response to a cue and substituting another behavior.

If you foresee a problem, for example, if you are going to a party where you will be exposed to temptation, recruit a friend to remind you of your goal (again, tactfully and gently!).

Plan Reinforcers

Plan reinforcers for positive behavior change and be specific about what you must do to earn them. Many behavior changes do have intrinsic rewards; however, sometimes these rewards are not immediate. The compliments from others and the healthy feelings you gain from exercise may not come during the first week of your program, when you have the most need for reinforcement. However, you can plan your own reinforcers. As Watson and Tharp (1981) state: "The best reinforcers are potent, accessible, and easily manipulatable by you." However, don't make these reinforcers so indispensable that you won't be willing to give them up if you don't do the required behavior to get them. You can flash on a quick mental image of yourself as you'll be when you've attained your goal. Give yourself lots of inner pats on the back and self-praise. You can do this immediately upon performing the behavior: "Good for me! I did it!"

Make sure that the total amount of reinforcement will be greater if you follow your behavior change program than if you don't. For example, if you always go out to dinner or a movie each week anyway, don't make those your only rewards; add some new ones. Your rewards should be small, frequent, and inexpensive ones, like a bunch of flowers or a movie. It is self-defeating to reward yourself with the very behavior you are trying to change, so avoid giving yourself an ice cream cone for a treat if you are attempting to follow a healthier diet.

Some people use tokens or a point system for reinforcing their positive behavior; this helps you bridge the gap between the behavior and the reward and allows you to give larger, more meaningful rewards to yourself on a less frequent basis while still getting an immediate positive reinforcer. You may decide to "up the ante" as you go, by requiring more advanced steps in your program to earn the reward. For example, during the first week of a weight loss program, reward yourself for keeping baseline records; during the second week reward yourself for cutting down on fats and increasing vegetables; during the third week earn the reward by adding some exercise as you continue the new diet. Always start with small, easy steps. Nothing succeeds like success!

Another important reinforcer for behavior change is social support. People can support you by joining you in exercising, quitting smoking, or eating vegetarian meals. Friends can praise or reward you for the positive steps you are taking. Please note that having people scold or punish you is NOT helpful; nor is it useful to do this to yourself if you slip up or fall back into an old behavior pattern. Finally, plan for some variety in the rewards so that you will stay motivated and not get bored. (A man who was using raisins for rewards found that they no longer inspired him by the third week.)

Plan Ahead for Relapses

Plan what you'll do if you relapse into the old behavior. Pronouncing yourself a failure and quitting is counterproductive. A better approach is to expect some relapses and have a plan to start over immediately with appropriate self-talk such as, "One slip doesn't negate all the good progress I've made; I can pick up where I left off. Each day is a new beginning." Ask yourself what happened and learn from the experience (e.g., a dieter might find that parties or Thanksgiving dinner are a problem for a diet and require special preparation). Be gentle with yourself. Have mercy! Self-acceptance, not self-control, is the key to positive change and healing.

Instructions

Describe your specific goal, plan of action, and an analysis of the advantages/disadvantages of your problem on the **Worksheet: Self-Healing Project Plan: Practice 14.**

Name _____ Date _____

Worksheet Self-Healing Project Plan: Practice 14

Problem or area of concern: _____

List the advantages and disadvantages of the behavior/problem you are planning to change.

Advantages	Disadvantages
_____	_____
_____	_____
_____	_____
_____	_____
_____	_____
_____	_____

STRATEGY AND PLAN OF ACTION

1. Goal and subgoals; criteria for success: _____

_____

_____

_____

_____

_____

2. Data collection plan: _____

_____

_____

_____

_____

_____

_____

_____

3. Social support: _____

_____

_____

_____

_____

4. Imagery use: _____

_____

5. Rewards and other reinforcers to make this project fun: _____

_____

_____

_____

6. Other aspects of your plan: _____

_____

_____

_____

_____

_____

_____

_____

_____

_____

_____

_____

Baseline measures:

Objective:_____

_____

Subjective:_____

_____

_____

IMAGERY FOR SELF-HEALING

Imagery is the mechanism by which will becomes effortless.

For some people, daily relaxation and imagery will be their main focus; for others, imagery may be a useful adjunct for effecting the behavior changes they have outlined after the practice of **imagery exploration.** In general, a blend of imagery and behavior change is most helpful. If you ignore an imagery message that guides you to make a change in your behavior, you may experience a sense of being stuck and may fail to make further progress. The underlying assumption is that mind/body/spirit are an integrated whole. Therefore, imagery can affect the body, promote healing, and enhance performance. Self-healing imagery can be helpful for virtually any somatic complaint.

Imagery may be either a primary or a complementary strategy for healing. In this way, with or without other treatments, you become an active participant in your healing process. This approach has been utilized in the treatment of cancer patients (Simonton, Matthews-Simonton, & Creighton, 1978). An effective imagery strategy consists of three components: inspecting the problem, illness, or area of discomfort; creating and experiencing an ongoing healing process that prevents relapses from occurring; and, finally, perceiving yourself whole and integrated. After having practiced this imagery draw or paint your area of concern in either anatomic or symbolic form, whichever came to you in your imagery experience. Also draw the healing process and yourself as you will be when completely whole, healed, and integrated. These drawings can be done several times and may change over the weeks. In this way they can provide a *before* and *after* measurement of inner change.

Imagery may also be used as an adjunct to behavior change. In this case the imagery is practiced as a form of mental rehearsal (as described in **Transforming Failure into Success: Practice 10).** For example, a man reported that it was much easier for him to go running in the morning if he first took a few minutes in bed picturing himself jogging briskly, enjoying the crisp morning air, and feeling how smoothly his muscles moved. Imaging worked both as a motivator and as a way to stay mindful of breathing and letting go of unneeded muscle tension.

Often, imagery is paired with activity. The more easily the healing imagery can be incorporated into little routines in your daily life, the more likely it is that it will always be present in the background of your activities. For example, several people reported that they used imagery while doing various forms of exercise and that they found it helped their endurance and enjoyment. One jogger pictured his higher self slightly ahead of him, drawing him onward. A woman who was visualizing the healing of an infection drank a glass of water before each visualization practice and then urinated afterward to dramatize ridding her body of the infection. Another person visualized shaking negative feelings (anger, anxiety) out of her body and into the earth while shaking her arms and legs out.

Concepts that Underlie Self-Healing Imagery

For 30 years my body has done its best to attract the attention of my conscious self.
                                                                    STUDENT

1. All areas of distress or illness are the body/mind's attempts to give us some important information to help us get back on our life's path. As one student reported:

> I had a dream in which I was riding a beautiful horse that was following a well-marked trail. Suddenly, my legs went into a spasm and squeezed the horse, forcing him to the right. Immediately, I felt embarrassed and got off the horse. He reared up and then looked me very sternly in the eye as though saying, "It's not okay for you to do that! I was on the path!" I take this to represent my mental tension pushing my physical being off the path.

So our task in imagery is to pay attention and get the message the symptom is trying to convey to us.

2. The person and the illness are separate. Imagery is meant to mobilize the higher self or the more creative aspects of the self. You are not your illness; the core of you is healthy.

3. The simple act of imaging a healing mechanism, which implies activity, will shift the sense of helplessness to a sense of control. Even if the healing mechanism makes no biological sense, simply conceiving of a tool for change is empowering. If you are receiving medical treatments concurrently, you may imagine them working in cooperation with your own healing process.

4. Include an image of wholeness or integration, even if complete physical recovery is not always possible. It is as valuable to mobilize a sense of wholeness/integration in a person who will never be physically healthy as it is to mobilize a sense of wellness in a person who has the biological possibility of becoming well. The image of wholeness/integration creates a sense of hope or possibility. Often, a diagnosis implies an internal, stable, and global situation. Patients often perceive their illness as their fault, lasting forever, and affecting all aspects of their life. The situation then feels hopeless, and change appears impossible. By imaging a mechanism for change and a new situation where there is no illness or problem, the internal, global, and stable concepts are changed. As you describe your images, note language that implies these attitudes and experiment with reframing the images by changing the descriptive language.

5. Letting go of the initial image that represents the illness or symptoms creates a possibility. Letting go of the image is difficult, especially when there is a significant amount of emotional experiences connected to the symptom. The tendency is to either hold on to the image or to aggressively throw it away. Ideally, you want to encourage a passive-attentional attitude toward the image; for example: "I notice this image and it is interesting, and I am not invested in it or attached to it." Surprisingly, this attitude of passive acceptance and open exploration allows the image to shift and change.

6. The imagery may change as the problem/illness changes. Always inspect your problem as it is RIGHT NOW. If you are truly in the present, you will see the problem/illness somewhat differently each time you inspect it. For example, if you

have a broken leg, at first the image may be similar to the X ray you saw at the doctor's office. The tendency is to keep this same mental picture of the X ray each time the imagery exercise is done. In reality, the body continuously changes. Hence, you need to be aware of the body's progress and observe changes each time. These changes may be subtle or drastic. In order to mobilize the self-healing potential, the images must be of the current state of affairs. As the inspected image changes, the healing mechanism will also have to change in order to be appropriate and useful with the new image of your problem area.

7. The goal is for the inspection and maintenance of a healing mechanism to become a constant background activity. Like humming a favorite song, imagery can occur in the back of consciousness at all times. It will take some time and understanding of the concepts before this type of integration takes place. The ultimate goal is to continually reassess and imagine the healing taking place, to feel the healing occurring. Many times throughout the day you will be touching with awareness and love that part of you which is ill or in pain.

8. Provide adequate time for relaxation, especially when you are first beginning your imagery practice. Images flow most easily into a relaxed mind.

9. Whatever image comes up, no matter how bizarre, illogical, or biologically incorrect, is the image to work with in the exercise. Our subconscious often accesses very important information for us through our images. These images may seem to make no sense; they may, however, be metaphors for some element involved in our condition. They may be very useful, especially as they relate to past events in our lives. Trust these images.

10. The healing mechanism must make sense within the imagery. The healing is not magic. There must be a logical transition between the problem area as it is at this moment and as it is when you are well or whole. The transition does not need to be realistic or literally possible, but it must make sense. The healing process must be stronger than the disease process. For example, if a person images his or her asthma as a brick wall and the healing mechanism as a magical swirl of light that suddenly creates a clear space, the healing mechanism becomes magical, rather than something over which the individual might have some control. A better image might include a bulldozer breaking the wall down and workers carrying the debris away and permanently disposing of it.

11. Explore associations to the image. It is important to understand what the image represents to *you*. Some images are universal or archetypal while others may have very personal and individual meanings.

12. Create a process by which the illness/problem can not return. For example, a woman with asthma imaged cleansing all the pollens from her lungs. The final step in the process was putting up a mesh screen so that the pollens could not enter in the future. (This could be a metaphor for the activation of the cilia, whose function is to sweep particulates from the airways.)

13. Externalize your image; that is, represent it in a physical form. This serves several purposes. In making the image tangible, it becomes changeable. It also separates the image from the person. Young children express their images in three dimensions as they play with their friends. Adults need help accessing their images in a form with which they can work comfortably. The following techniques, among others, can be used to externalize the image. Use these techniques not just once but

several times over the course of your self-healing program; in this way you can gain added insights and also see changes in your images over time.

- Draw or paint three different images illustrating the area of concern as it is at this moment, the healing process, and health, wholeness, or integration. If drawing or painting feels difficult, try a collage of images you select from magazines. It is helpful to do the visual representation before writing or talking about the image.
- Describe the images verbally to others. The image will often tend to stay on an intellectual level if it is just thought about.
- Model the three images out of clay. This may be more comfortable than drawing for some people.
- Imagine spontaneous sounds or select three musical compositions that represent the images. For example, one woman described her back pain like steak sizzling on a grill. Another woman, working with depression, selected depressing music, neutral music, and joyful music; she also began humming and singing the joyful music.
- Act out the images physically; you may even involve others. For example, one or more people could represent the area of concern and others could play the part of the healing mechanism as the imager directs the play.
- Take pictures with a camera that represent the images you saw in your inspection and healing process. This technique is useful for people who find it difficult to express their images using any of the other modalities. A Polaroid camera works best.
- Take a walk and find flowers, rocks, clouds, and so on that symbolize the images.

Examples of Self-Healing Imagery

A woman with carpal tunnel syndrome described the self-healing imagery process as follows:

> My experience with the self-healing image dramatically changed from the first vision of pain to one of healing. At first my hand was gray and cold. I felt aching pain in the wrist and fingers of my right hand. When visualizing health, at first only the fingertips of my hand were changed in color to a reddish hue. Eventually, as the exercise progressed, my entire hand became physically warm with a pleasant feeling of free-flowing blood and nerves transmitting through the wrist to the tips of my fingers. My entire hand took on a reddish glow. This image became the final image of health—one I found I could easily bring into focus. . . .I found when I followed my self-healing recommendations—wearing my splint at night, being aware of muscle fatigue and consciously relieving it through muscle relaxation, and exercising the self-healing imagery—my hand became asymptomatic. However, if I deviated from this schedule, as I did a few times, the symptoms returned. My awareness of muscle fatigue has become more automatic in most activities involving my hand.

A competitive tennis player who had twisted her ankle 2 weeks before a scheduled tournament imaged blood cells and lymph flowing to and from her ankle and calcium being brought for the tendons to grow. Her ankle healed, and she played in the tournament.

A student with back pain saw "an image of a brick mason trying to patch up a hole in a wall." As she tried to see what was behind the wall, a sentry appeared to guard it. "A big wave of fear came over me. It really scared me that there was something so powerful hidden behind that wall and that it was trying to burst out." As she continued with the imagery, she reported, "I saw the pain as a sharp thorn in my back which was blocking the flow of energy." As she directed the free flow of energy, she saw her chest "opening up in the front so that the pain did not need to push out the back." She tried to visualize the removal of the thorn: "I realized that the thorn was my husband, and I couldn't pull it out. Although we had been separated for almost a year, I had put off getting a divorce. The fear I was feeling was fear of my unknown future. Rather than face an uncertain future, I was keeping that tie to my husband even though it was causing me pain." As she began to let go of the past, she was able to pull the thorn out a little. "I saw the tip of the thorn break off inside me and I felt it bloom into something wonderful. I felt that meant that the good things I had gotten from my marriage would continue to stay with me and I could let the rest go." While she continued using visualization, movement, and sound, she filed for a divorce, and the pain diminished greatly in 4 weeks.

A man began the process of shrinking his wart by imagining a tiny warrior shooting lasers at it. He wrote:

> Philosophically speaking at least, the last thing anyone needs is more violent imagery. And further, there is no telling what sorts of negative effects such imagery has on the body or mind, even when the intended outcome is achieved. One thing I would like to try instead would be to visualize a negotiated settlement with the virus in question. Maybe I could get the virus to pack up his wart and leave.

He was able to modify his imagery in order to become more comfortable with it.

Some people have complex and biologically correct images while others see abstract and/or simple images. One man with chronic hepatitis and gastrointestinal distress, who happened to have a strong background in biology, integrated relaxation and visualization every day: Picturing himself to be very small, he would imagine going inside his liver and watching the hepatitis viruses replicate. He could see the white cells eat the virus particles after they had burst from the liver cells where they had replicated. He also saw some of the viruses enter new liver cells, where they continued to replicate and which they caused to burst. What he imaged for 3 months was the perfect model to maintain the status quo, namely, a picture of white cells destroying some of the virus particles while others were free to invade more healthy liver cells. There was no mechanism in his model to prevent the liver cells from being infected by the virus. In his new image, the man saw himself painting his liver cells with a protective chemical that would prevent the virus from attacking the healthy cells. Now his white cells could make progress instead of simply preventing things from getting worse, and within a month his liver functions were normal. It is essential that the healing mechanism being imaged contain a protective component or create a permanent change in the illness so that it cannot come back.

There is no right way to experience an image. Respect whatever images you have in whatever forms they come to you, as they will most likely provide you with valuable information. And be willing to allow new images to replace images that are not working for you.

NOTE: When making your own tape, substitute your personal relaxation script (Practice 8) in place of the indented sample script.

Relaxation and Self-Healing Imagery Script

Wiggle around and make yourself comfortable . . . Loosen any constricting clothing; loosen your collar, take off your glasses, take off your watch, and remove your wallet and keys from your pocket (if you wear hard contacts, you might want to take them out as it is difficult to relax the eyes with them in) . . . Be sure your belt, upper buttons, and upper 2 inches of your pants zipper are loose. Sit comfortably in a chair or lie comfortably on a sofa or bed (when lying down, make sure you have a pillow beneath your knees and under your head).

Insert your personal relaxation script (Practice 8) or use the following sample relaxation script.

Now close your eyes and slowly scan your body. If you notice any place that feels uncomfortable, tighten that area and let it go. . . Scan your whole body from the top of your head to the tips of your toes—face, neck, and shoulders; lower back, arms, and hands; chest, stomach, and buttocks; legs, feet, and toes. Now lift your hands slightly from your lap and make a fist with both hands . . . Feel the tightness in your arms while you keep breathing . . . Be sure that the rest of your body stays relaxed. Feel the tension in your arms; let go and relax . . . Feel the relaxation flowing down your arms and out your hands.

Now, while breathing and keeping your neck and jaw relaxed, raise your shoulders to your ears . . . Feel the tightness in your upper chest and shoulders. Let go and relax . . . Feel the relaxation flowing down your shoulders and arms like an ocean wave. Now curl your toes up as you press your heels down . . . While feeling the tightness in your legs, be sure that you are breathing and that your jaw, neck, and shoulders are relaxed. . . Let go and relax . . . Imagine a wave of relaxation going down your legs and out your feet . . . Feel your body relaxing and let your breathing become slower . . . and . . . slower.

Let the air move easily in and out like an ocean wave . . . Be sure to exhale by gently pulling your stomach in at the end of the exhalation. When you inhale allow your abdomen to expand and widen. Let your breath flow easily in and out, in and out.

As you inhale, imagine that you can feel the air coming through your feet into your ankles, calves, knees, thighs, and buttocks . . . As you exhale, imagine the air flowing down your arms and legs and out your fingers and toes . . . Imagine the air going outward forever, flowing down your arms and legs and out your hands and feet . . . As you exhale, imagine the warmth flowing down and outward . . . Let each breath be slower and longer . . . Let your breath slow down . . . If your attention wanders, let the distraction be a reminder to breathe slowly and regularly while feeling the air going down your arms and legs . . . Become aware of the throbbing of the pulse in the fingers . . . Feel the hands warming as the breath moves down and through the arms . . . Continue breathing easily for the next few minutes.

After completing your personal relaxation script, or the sample script, continue with the following script.

The more you practice, the easier it becomes and the easier it is to reach a deeper awareness that allows you to mobilize your self-healing potential and become whole . . . The more you practice, the more you will know that you are mobilizing your own health potential. . .

Let your breathing slow down and deepen. . . As the breath flows calmly and regularly, continue to repeat your own phrase (such as "I am at peace"). . . For the next few minutes allow your attention to go with your breathing while you continue to repeat your phrase . . . Let your breathing become slower and deeper . . . As your breath slows down, know that you are mobilizing your health.

Now let go of the phrase and allow your breath to continue slowly and evenly . . . Begin to inspect your area of concern. . . Just look and feel inside to see what this area looks like at this moment in time . . . Allow any image, sensation, or thought to occur. The image may be in black and white or in color or it may be a bodily sensation or an emotion . . . Whatever occurs, let it be.

Now let go of that image. . . Imagine a process by which healing and wholeness occur, a process that transforms what you saw during the inspection into health and wholeness . . . See and feel the healing process . . . For the next few minutes allow the healing process to continue.

The healing process continues all the time: it is often beneath our awareness, yet it continues. For some, it becomes like a musical melody that we hum in the back of our heads all day long . . . Feel the healing being carried through to completion . . . Let a single image or symbol come to you that you can hold in your mind throughout the day.

Now shift your imagery and experience yourself whole and integrated . . . Know that you are part of the universe . . . Experience a deep, gentle quietness . . . Allow the breath to move easily in and out . . . in and out. Imagine that as you inhale, a healing energy comes into you like the rays of the sun, penetrating every cell with a shimmering light, and as you exhale, the healing energy spreads outward like a blue cloud or wave . . . Allow this process to continue for a few minutes . . . See yourself joyously moving through your day, doing the things you love to do, enjoying just being yourself, feeling free and content.

After a few minutes, continue with the next section.

Remember, each time you practice you are mobilizing your self-healing potential. . . Congratulate yourself for enhancing your own wholeness and health and allow the healing process and healing energy to continue to flow through you during the day.

You can choose to become more aware of the present environment or allow yourself to fall asleep . . . If you want to get up, take a deep breath, feeling relaxed yet alert, then gently open your eyes while stretching your arms . . . Whether asleep or awake, be aware that the healing process continues all the time.

Each day after you have gone through the script, describe your experience on the **Log Sheet: Practice 14** and draw the images of the problem area, the healing process, and wholeness/integration. When you describe your healing imagery, be sure that the healing mechanism is concrete and not "magical" and that the problem has been permanently changed so that it cannot return. The drawings will reflect the multidimensionality of the images. They may range from a simple black blob to a very complex biological rendition of the lungs or a multicolored abstract picture. These are all equally valid images.

CARRYING OUT AND ADAPTING YOUR STRATEGY: PRACTICE 14

You might decide to write up a contract specifying what you plan to do and then sign it. You may also ask a good friend or family member to cosign it. This helps you solidify your commitment. Carry out your strategy, keeping log notes on your self-devised log forms. Evaluate your strategy as you go, making changes when appropriate. Sometimes a strategy that looks perfect on paper will reveal a few flaws as you put it into practice; in fact, it is nearly impossible to construct a perfect strategy for self-healing without having to make modifications somewhere along the line. You may discover new information in your readings that you will want to incorporate. You may realize that it is because your data collection system is too cumbersome that you aren't doing it; a simplification of your system may be all you need to get back on track.

Continue to keep progress notes throughout your behavior change project. Making graphs and charts can show satisfying evidence of changes and can also help you troubleshoot. If you're not progressing as you'd like, find out what's getting in the way and revise your program. People often set subgoals that are too big. If jogging is your plan, starting with a quarter mile may be too ambitious, especially if you've been sedentary. Perhaps you need to start with walking around the block for the first week. Perhaps you need more enticing rewards—or prompter ones. Do you have the social support you need? Are you using mental rehearsal to practice the new behaviors before you go into them?

Each day after you have gone through the script, complete **Log Sheet: Practice 14 (Week 1).** At the end of the week, answer **Questions: Practice 14 (Week 1).** Then review your experience by answering the **Questions for Reflection: Practice 14.** From that analysis, adapt your self-healing strategy and outline any changes you plan to make. Finally, meet with your group and complete **Discussions and Conclusions: Practice 14.**

Use the information from **Discussion and Conclusions: Practice 14** and **Questions for Reflection: Practice 14** to fine-tune your self-healing practice. Continue these practices for the next 3 weeks. Each day complete the appropriate **Log Sheet: Practice 14** and then review your experience through **Questions for Reflection: Practice 14** and meet with your group and complete the **Discussion and Conclusion: Practice 14** worksheet for the week.

Name _____ Date _____

Log Sheet Self-Healing: Practice 14 (Week 1)

Each day (a) describe your experience with your self-healing practice and (b) record the objective and/or subjective data. You may need to use your self-devised data sheets here.

Day 1   a. _____

Date _____   _____

_____

_____

           b. _____

_____

_____

_____

Day 2   a. _____

Date _____   _____

_____

_____

           b. _____

_____

_____

_____

Day 3   a. _____

Date _____   _____

_____

_____

           b. _____

_____

_____

_____

Day 4   a. _____
Date _____   _____
_____
_____
              b. _____
_____
_____
_____

Day 5   a. _____
Date _____   _____
_____
_____
              b. _____
_____
_____
_____

Day 6   a. _____
Date _____   _____
_____
_____
              b. _____
_____
_____
_____

Day 7   a. _____
Date _____   _____
_____
_____
              b. _____
_____
_____

Name _____ Date _____

Questions Self-Healing: Practice 14 (Week 1)

1. What benefits occurred as a result of your practice?

_____
_____
_____
_____
_____

2. How did your mood and physical state change before, during, and after the practices?

_____
_____
_____
_____

3. What changes did you observe in your objective/subjective data?

_____
_____
_____
_____
_____

4. How will you change or adapt the practice for next week to enhance your success?

_____
_____
_____
_____

5. What problems/challenges occurred and how did you solve them?

_____
_____
_____
_____

Discussion and Conclusions   Self-Healing: Practice 14 (Week 1)

1. What benefits and successes did the group members notice as a result of the practice?

_____

_____

_____

_____

2. How are your group members valuable resources in helping you brainstorm ideas to adapt your strategy?

_____

_____

_____

3. How do levels of commitment relate to achieving small successes in this first week? How did the rewards influence your practice?

_____

_____

_____

4. What are some creative ways by which group members monitor their behavior?

_____

_____

_____

_____

5. Topics for which instructor consultation would be helpful:

_____

_____

_____

List your group members: _____ _____

_____ _____ _____

_____ _____ _____

Questions for Reflection   Self-Healing: Practice 14[3]

____ How high is my level of commitment to my self-healing?
____ Am I clear about my goal and subgoals?
____ Do I need to change or modify any of these?
____ Are they expressed in measurable behavioral terms?
____ Have I broken down my strategy into small manageable chunks?
____ Did I establish a clear baseline?
____ How well did my self-devised log forms work for my data collection so far? What could I do to improve them?
____ Am I keeping consistent written records? If not, why not?
____ Do I need assistance in monitoring my behavior? How could I get it?
____ What's getting in my way? What are my excuses, and how can I talk myself out of them?
____ Have I carefully examined the advantages of changing and compared them with the advantages of not changing?
____ How helpful is my inner language? Can I improve it?
____ Have I asked for, and received, social support for carrying out my plans? If not, why not?
____ Have I given myself positive reinforcement, or small rewards, for getting started on my project? If not, why not?
____ How effective were my reinforcers in motivating me?
____ How could I involve others in reinforcing me?
____ Am I using mental rehearsal to help me develop new behavior?
____ Have I incorporated insights from imagery into my strategy?
____ Am I keeping my sense of humor about it all?
____ ARE WE HAVING FUN YET? (If it isn't fun, why bother???)

OUTLINE ANY CHANGES YOU PLAN TO MAKE IN YOUR STRATEGY:

_____

_____

_____

_____

_____

_____

_____

Name _____ Date _____

Log Sheet Self-Healing: Practice 14 (Week 2)

Each day describe your experience with your self-healing practice and record the objective and/or subjective data. You may need to use your self-devised data sheets here.

Day 1   a. _____
Date _____   _____
                _____
                _____
             b. _____
                _____
                _____
                _____

Day 2   a. _____
Date _____   _____
                _____
             b. _____
                _____
                _____
                _____

Day 3   a. _____
Date _____   _____
                _____
             b. _____
                _____
                _____
                _____

Day 4   a. _____
Date _____   _____

_____

_____

b. _____

_____

_____

_____

Day 5   a. _____
Date _____   _____

_____

_____

b. _____

_____

_____

_____

Day 6   a. _____
Date _____   _____

_____

_____

b. _____

_____

_____

_____

Day 7   a. _____
Date _____   _____

_____

_____

b. _____

_____

_____

Name _____ Date _____

Questions   Self-Healing: Practice 14 (Week 2)

1. What benefits occurred as a result of your practice?

_____

_____

_____

_____

_____

2. What changes did you observe in your objective/subjective data?

_____

_____

_____

_____

3. How did you reward/reinforce yourself for doing the practices?

_____

_____

_____

_____

4. What changes did you experience within your imagery?

_____

_____

_____

5. How will you change or adapt the practice for next week to enhance your success?

_____

_____

_____

_____

_____

Name_____ Date_____

Discussion and Conclusions   Self-Healing: Practice 14 (Week 2)

1. What benefits and successes did the group members notice as a result of the practice?

_____
_____
_____
_____
_____
_____

2. What are some creative ways by which group members monitor their behavior?

_____
_____
_____
_____
_____
_____

3. What was the role of imagery in achieving a positive change?

_____
_____
_____
_____
_____

4. Topics for which instructor consultation would be helpful:

_____
_____

List your group members: _____ _____
_____ _____ _____
_____ _____ _____

Name _____ Date _____

Log Sheet   Self-Healing: Practice 14 (Week 3)

Each day (a) describe your experience with your self-healing practice and {b) record the objective and/or subjective data. (You may use your own log forms instead.)

Day 1   a. _____

Date _____   _____

_____

_____

              b. _____

_____

_____

_____

Day 2   a. _____

Date _____   _____

_____

_____

              b. _____

_____

_____

_____

Day 3   a. _____

Date _____   _____

_____

_____

              b. _____

_____

_____

_____

Day 4   a. _____
Date _____   _____
               _____
               _____
               b. _____
               _____
               _____
               _____

Day 5   a. _____
Date _____   _____
               _____
               b. _____
               _____
               _____
               _____

Day 6   a. _____
Date _____   _____
               _____
               b. _____
               _____
               _____
               _____

Day 7   a. _____
Date _____   _____
               _____
               b. _____
               _____
               _____
               _____

Name _____ Date _____

Questions   Self-Healing: Practice 14 (Week 3)

1. What benefits occurred as a result of your practice?

_____

_____

_____

_____

2. What changes did you observe in your objective/subjective data?

_____

_____

_____

_____

3. How are you using your log sheets as feedback to help you change your behavior?

_____

_____

_____

_____

4. What social support are you receiving and is it helpful?

_____

_____

_____

5. How will you change or adapt the practice for next week to enhance your success?

_____

_____

_____

Name_____ Date_____

Discussion and Conclusions   Self-Healing: Practice 14 (Week 3)

1. What benefits and successes did the group members notice as a result of the practice?

_____

_____

_____

_____

_____

_____

2. What are some creative ways by which group members monitor and reward their behavior?

_____

_____

_____

_____

_____

_____

3. How did social support help or hinder behavior change among group members?

_____

_____

_____

_____

_____

4. Topics for which instructor consultation would be helpful:

_____

_____

List your group members: _____ _____

_____ _____ _____

_____ _____ _____

Name _____ Date _____

Log Sheet Self-Healing: Practice 14 (Week 4)

Each day describe (a) your experience with your self-healing practice and (b) record the objective and/or subjective data (you may use your own log forms instead).

Day 1   a. _____
Date _____   _____
_____
_____

            b. _____
_____
_____
_____

Day 2   a. _____
Date _____   _____
_____
_____

            b. _____
_____
_____
_____

Day 3   a. _____
Date _____   _____
_____
_____

            b. _____
_____
_____
_____

Day 4   a. _____

Date _____   _____

_____

_____

             b. _____

_____

_____

_____

Day 5   a. _____

Date _____   _____

_____

_____

             b. _____

_____

_____

_____

Day 6   a. _____

Date _____   _____

_____

_____

             b. _____

_____

_____

_____

Day 7   a. _____

Date _____   _____

_____

_____

             b. _____

_____

_____

Name _____ Date _____

Questions Self-Healing: Practice 14 (Week 4)

1. What benefits occurred as a result of your practice?

_____

_____

_____

_____

_____

_____

2. What changes did you observe in your objective/subjective data?

_____

_____

_____

_____

_____

3. How are you using inner language/self-talk to support your behavior change/self-healing?

_____

_____

_____

_____

4. How will you integrate the self-healing practices into your daily life from this time on?

_____

_____

_____

_____

_____

Discussion and Conclusions   Self-Healing: Practice 14 (Week 4)

1. What benefits and successes did the group members notice as a result of the practice?

_____
_____
_____
_____
_____

2. What are some creative ways by which group members monitor and reward their behavior?

_____
_____
_____
_____
_____

3. How will the group members continue to integrate their self-healing strategies into their daily lives?

_____
_____
_____
_____
_____
_____

4. Topics for which instructor consultation would be helpful:

_____
_____

List your group members: _____ _____
_____ _____ _____
_____ _____ _____

INTEGRATING YOUR EXPERIENCE

Integrating what you experienced by summarizing what you learned and writing up your results can enhance the self-healing process. Write about your experience as suggested in the section "Reflection and Integration: Summarizing Your Experience" at the end of Chapter 1. Reflect over the last weeks, reread your logs, and gently ask yourself the following questions: How did this self-healing process change me? What did I learn from this? How did I grow? Respect both the setbacks (or challenges) and the successes. Your self-report is a testament to change, as some of the following reports indicate.

Report 1: Weight and Self-Image

My body did change during my practice. I lost a total of 3 pounds and 7.5 inches from my body. My inner sense of my body also changed. As the weeks continued, my blimp became smaller and smaller. The blimp is still there, but it has decreased from being about the size of a whale to about the size of a very small fish (see Figure 4.1). My feelings that were buried beneath my obsession with my weight also became uncovered. My sensuality is related to my obsession. I am afraid to become close with any man, and yet I long for the intimacy. I have been in a committed relationship for 5 years, yet I feel extreme ambivalence about the relationship. During the past few weeks, as I have confronted my own fears of intimacy, the ambivalence has lessened. Not only have I become a little lighter in body weight but my emotional weight has decreased.

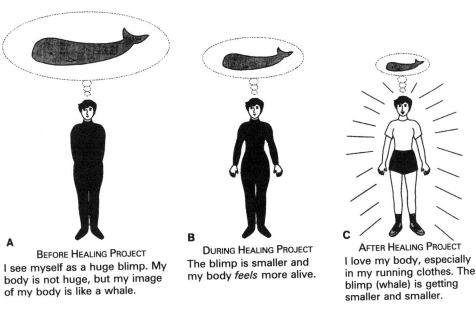

A
BEFORE HEALING PROJECT
I see myself as a huge blimp. My body is not huge, but my image of my body is like a whale.

B
DURING HEALING PROJECT
The blimp is smaller and my body *feels* more alive.

C
AFTER HEALING PROJECT
I love my body, especially in my running clothes. The blimp (whale) is getting smaller and smaller.

FIGURE 4.1. Self-image change during healing process.

Report 2: Physical Exercise

When I began this project, my focus was on physical exercise and creating a mental image of the body that I would like to have. My project carried me to places deep inside myself that I didn't know existed. I realized that body weight was an obsession. Beneath this obsessiveness was a layer of fear and rage. I feared being sensual and felt rage that I really wanted to be desirable. I have not gotten through this yet, but this was the beginning of uncovering the layers of feelings that have run my life for 20 years. In addition, I felt the power of using visualization while running. My running distance doubled and I enjoyed my running more than ever before. Something inside me opened to feel the energy of life flow through me. I felt connected with my body. I began to get a glimpse of grace.

Report 3: Mood Swings

In my imagery, at first I saw myself on top of a beautiful green hill. There was a swing set at the apex and I got on it. As I swung out I saw a beautiful valley with three different roads all leading off into the horizon; ... but when the swing came down, it was as if I had lost sight of this beautiful valley and it was too much to bear. I decided to get off the swing. ... This allowed me to see that possibilities stretched on forever. Getting off the swing in this visualization made me feel that I had made a conscious decision to do so in my life as well. Once I had a clear view of this valley, I realized that there weren't three roads after all. There was really only one, on which it was possible to go off on a confusing side road—or go too fast and get out of control if one was not careful. I worked with this visualization as a 20-minute meditation every morning for about two weeks. I realized that there was a car on this road and that the driver of the car was not me (I was only the passenger). I changed this arrangement. . . .

I was surprised to find that I didn't need the full 20 minutes every morning to have this imagery work for me. I was also using this imagery for quick adjustments throughout the day. If I was feeling harried or down, I would close my eyes and look at the car on the road. Was I going too fast? I would take my foot off the accelerator a bit. What was causing me to be disagreeable? If I was tired, I would rest; if hungry, I would eat. . . .

This self-healing strategy feels very successful . . . I had a couple of occasions in which I was more out of control than I wanted to be . . . By summoning up my imagery I was able to see what was happening to me. I then quickly apologized and tried to explain the situation to whomever I had offended. In this way, then, a mood wasn't able to get further out of control. Most of my ups and downs were stabilized within minutes. . . . Another measure of success for me is that I was able to go through my PMS with only slight irritation and disorientation . . . what I thought was a completely chemical reaction going on in my body that I had no control over was something different. I could see that at least part of my symptoms were caused by my thoughts.

Observations of changes in a person that are made by others provide an even more dramatic testimonial to progress. The roommate of the woman just quoted reported as follows:

J. has always been an emotional person . . . her angry outbursts . . . have been venomous . . . . Her bouts of depression have been sad to witness, and at its worst [the depression] usually manifested itself by her staunch refusal to get out of bed. So there she would lie, all day, under the covers, feeling very pathetic. . . . These fluctuations . . . always seemed to be part of her nature. Something to be endured. . . .

[This self-healing program] has certainly had a profound effect on J. If mood swings were once sudden, unpredictable, and extremely wide-ranging, now—if they occur at all—they are controlled and very short-lived. The sense I get is that J. has become more centered. Rather than learning to simply control her mood swings, it seems J. has become a better person, a more peaceful and a stronger person, and so has become more stable and less inclined to exhibit the types of uncontrolled behavior usually associated with an unstable personality. She has become easier to deal with, and has also been able to deal with me in a more diplomatic way (and I am no Mother Theresa). The best part of all this is that J. has shared her wisdom gained in the last few weeks with me; so perhaps I have become a better person too.

SUGGESTED READINGS

Achterberg, J. (1985). *Imagery in Healing: Shamanism and Modern Medicine.* Boston: New Science Library.

Bresler, D. (1979). *Free Yourself from Pain.* New York: Simon & Schuster.

Capacchione, L. (1991). *Recovery of Your Inner Child.* New York: Simon & Schuster.

Fish, R., Weakland, J. H., & Segal, L. (1982). *The Tactics of Change.* San Francisco: Jossey-Bass.

Frank, A. W. (1991). *At the Will of the Body.* Boston: Houghton Mifflin.

King, S. (1981). *Imagineering for Health.* Wheaton, IL: Theosophical Publishing House.

Norris, P. & Porter, G. (1985). *I Choose Life.* Walpole, NH: Stillpoint.

Robin, E. D. (1984). *Matters of Life and Death: Risk Versus Benefits of Medical Care.* New York: W. H. Freeman.

Rossman, M. L. (1987). *Healing Yourself.* New York: Walker.

Samuels, M. & Samuels, N. (1975). *Seeing with the Mind's Eye.* New York: Random House.

Simonton, O. C., Matthews-Simonton, S., & Creighton, J. L. (1978). *Getting Well Again.* New York: Bantam Books.

Watson, D. L. & Tharp, R. G. (1981). *Self-Directed Behavior: Self-Modification for Personal Adjustment.* Monterey: Brooks/Cole.

Watzlawick, P., Weakland, J., & Fisch, R. (1974). *Change.* New York:

Appendix
Audiotapes and Temperature Monitoring Devices

Audiotapes of the practices and temperature-monitoring devices (cards and thermometers) can be ordered from:

Breathing for Health
2236 Derby Street
Berkeley, CA 94705
TEL: (510)841-7227 FAX: (510)658-9801

Temperature monitoring devices: Temperature cards (about $2.00 and similar to the card enclosed in this workbook) and hand-held alcohol thermometers (about $1.00) can be ordered from:

SPC Center, Inc.
11949 Jefferson Boulevard, Suite 104
Culver City, CA 90230
TEL: (213)301-3317 FAX: (213)306-3917

American Biotechnology Corporation
24 Browning Drive
Ossining, NY 10562
TEL: (800)424-6832 FAX: (914)762-2281

Conscious Living Foundation
P.O. Box 9
Drain, OR
TEL: (503)836-2358

Stens Corporation
6451 Oakwood Drive
Oakland, CA 94611
TEL: (800)257-9053 FAX: (510)339-2222

Small portable electronic thermistors (about $50.00) can be ordered from:

American Biotechnology Corporation
24 Browning Drive
Ossining, NY 10562
TEL: (800)424-6832 FAX: (914)762-2281

Bio-Medical Instruments, Inc.
2387 E. 8 Mile Road
Warren, MI 48091-2403
TEL: (800)521-4640

Stens Corporation
6451 Oakwood Drive
Oakland, CA 94611
TEL: (800)257-8367 FAX: (510)339-2222

Thought Technology Ltd.
2180 Telgrave Avenue
Montreal, QU H4A 2L8
Canada
TEL: (800)361-3651 FAX: (514)489-8255

Notes

Chapter 1: Introduction

1. About 50% of who we are, including our personalities/temperament, is genetically determined.
2. See the Appendix for information on source of audiotapes for the practices.
3. Adapted from E. Peper and E. Williams, *From the Inside Out: A Self Teaching and Laboratory Manual for Biofeedback* (New York: Plenum, 1981).
4. See the Appendix for sources of audiotapes.

Chapter 2: Dynamic Relaxation

1. We borrowed the term *dynamic relaxation* from Joel Levey's book *The Fine Arts of Relaxation, Concentration and Meditation* (London: Wisdom, 1987).
2. During this exercise, or during later practice of dynamic relaxation, electromyographic (EMG) biofeedback may be helpful in confirming that other body parts are not being tightened.
3. Adapted from E. Peper, *Breathing for Health* (Montreal: Thought Technology, 1990).
4. Adapted from L. C. Lum, "The Syndrome of Habitual Chronic Hyperventilation," in *Modern Trends in Psychosomatic Medicine*, ed. V. Hill (London: Butterworth, 1976), pp. 196–230.
5. This anecdote was adapted from a talk by Theodore Melnechuk.
6. Adapted from C. F. Stroebel, *QR: The Quieting Reflex* (New York: Putnam, 1982).
7. Much of this early work is described in E. Green and A. Green, *Beyond Biofeedback* (New York: Delacorte, 1977).
8. See the Appendix for sources for additional temperature monitoring devices.
9. Adapted from N. Cousins, *Head First: The Biology of Hope* (New York: Dutton, 1989), pp. 89–88.

10. Adapted from C. F. Stroebel, *QR, The Quieting Reflex* (New York: Putnam, 1982).

Chapter 3: Cognitive Balance

1. For more detailed background, self-assessment, and strategies for change, read M. E. P. Seligman, *Learned Optimism* (New York: Knopf, 1991).
2. Adapted from the research of James Pennebaker. For more detailed descriptions, see J. W. Pennebaker, *Opening Up: The Healing Power of Confiding in Others* (New York: Morrow, 1991).

Chapter 4: Self-Healing Through Imagery and Behavior Change

1. The behavioral approaches have been adapted from D. Watson and R. Tharp, *Self-Directed Behavior: Self-Modification for Personal Adjustment* (Monterey, CA: Brooks/Cole, 1981). We recommend this text to anyone desiring to change their behavior.
2. For specific information, we recommend that you search relevant databases such as *Index Medicus* and *Psychological Abstracts*. Contact your reference librarian for more information. Most university libraries subscribe to these databases in printed form, compact disks, CD-ROM, or direct computer access.
3. Adapted from D. Watson and R. Tharp, *Self-Directed Behavior: Self-Modification for Personal Adjustment* (Monterey, CA: Brooks/Cole, 1981).

References

Ader, R. & Cohen, N. (1975). Behaviorally conditioned immunosuppression. *Psychosomatic Medicine, 37,* 333–340.

Bernstein, D. A. & Borkovec, T. (1973). *Progressive Relaxation Training: A Manual for the Helping Professions.* Champaign, IL: Research Press.

Cannon, W. B. (1939). *The Wisdom of the Body* (2nd ed.). New York: Norton.

Capacchione, L. (1988). *The Power of Your Other Hand.* North Hollywood, CA: Newcastle.

Capacchione, L. (1991). *Recovery of Your Inner Child.* New York: Simon & Schuster.

Chopra, D. (1989). *Quantum Healing:* New York. Bantam Books, p. 87.

Cousins, N. (1989). *Head First: The Biology of Hope.* New York: Dutton.

Ellis, A. (1979). The basic clinical theory of rational emotive therapy. In A. Ellis & M. M. Whitelay (Eds.), *Theoretical and Empirical Foundations of Rational-Emotive Therapy.* Monterey, CA: Brooks/Cole, pp. 33–60.

Fahrion, S., Norris, P., Green, A., Green, E., & Snarr, C. (1986). Biobehavioral treatment of essential hypertension: A group outcome study. *Biofeedback and Self-Regulation, 11,* 257–278.

Frank, A. W. (1991). *At the Will of the Body.* Boston: Houghton Mifflin.

Freedman, R. (1987). Long-term effectiveness of behavioral treatments for Raynaud's disease. *Behavior Therapy, 18,* 387–399.

Ghanta, V., Hiramoto, R., Solvason, H., & Spector, H. (1985). Neural and environmental influence on neoplasia and conditioning of natural killer cell activity. *Journal of Immunology, 135,* 848s–852s.

Green, E. E. & Green, A. M. (1977). *Beyond Biofeedback.* New York: Delacorte.

Hanh, T. N. (1976). *The Miracle of Mindfulness! A Manual on Meditation.* Boston: Beacon Press.

Hanna, T. (1988). *Somatics.* Reading, MA: Addison-Wesley.

Jacobson, E. (1970). *Modern Treatment of Tense Patients.* Springfield, IL: Thomas.

Jacobson, E. (1974). *Progressive Relaxation* (3rd ed.). Chicago: University of Chicago Press.

Jacobson, E. (1976). *You Must Relax.* New York: Whittlesey House.

Justice, B. (1988). *Who Gets Sick: How Beliefs, Moods and Thoughts Affect Your Health.* Los Angeles: Tarcher.

Kobasa, S. C., Maddi, S. R., & Kahn, S. (1982). Hardiness and health: A prospective study. *Journal of Personality and Social Psychology, 42*(1), 168–177.

Kung, Dora Van Gelder. (1991). *The Personal Aura.* Wheaton, IL: Quest Books.

Levey, J. & Levey, M. (1987). *The Fine Arts of Relaxation, Concentration, and Meditation.* Boston: Wisdom.

Levy, S. M. (1985). *Behavior and Cancer.* San Francisco: Jossey-Bass.

Lum, L. C. (1976). The syndrome of habitual chronic hyperventilation. In L. Hill (Ed.), *Modern Trends in Psychosomatic Medicine* (pp. 196–230). London: Butterworth.

Mackenzie, J. H. (1886). The production of the so-called "rose cold" by means of an artificial rose. *American Journal of Medical Science, 91,* 45–57.

McEwen, B. W. (1990). Hormones and the nervous system. *Advances, 7*(1), 50–54.

Meichenbaum, D. H. (1977). *Cognitive Behavior Modification.* New York: Plenum.

Norris, P. & Porter, G. (1987). *I Choose Life.* Walpole, NH: Stillpoint.

Palmer, S., Tibbetts, V., & Peper, E. (1991). The effects of self-willed unilateral vasodilation on the healing rates of bilateral wounds. *Proceedings of the Twenty-Second Annual Meeting of the Association for Applied Psychophysiology and Biofeedback* (pp. 124–127). Wheat Ridge, CO: AAPB.

Pelletier, K. R. (1977). *Mind as Healer, Mind as Slayer.* New York: Dell.

Pennebaker, J. W. (1991). *Opening Up: The Healing Power of Confiding in Others.* New York: Morrow.

Peper, E. (1990). *Breathing for Health.* Montreal: Thought Technology.

Peper, E. & Grossman, E. (1979). Thermal biofeedback training in children with headache. In E. Peper, S. Ancoli, & M. Quinn (Eds.), *Mind/Body Integration: Essential Readings in Biofeedback* (pp. 489–492). New York: Plenum.

Peper, E. & Williams, E. A. (1981). *From the Inside Out: A Self-Teaching and Laboratory Manual for Biofeedback.* New York: Plenum.

Rossman, M. L. (1987). *Healing Yourself.* New York: Walker.

Seligman, M. E. P. (1991). *Learned Optimism.* New York: Knopf.

Selye, H. (1956). *The Stress of Life.* New York: McGraw-Hill.

Selye, H. (1974). *Stress without Distress.* New York: Lippincott.

Simonton, O. C., Matthews-Simonton, S., & Creighton, J. L. (1978). *Getting Well Again.* New York: Bantam Books.

Stroebel, C. F. (1982) *QR: The Quieting Reflex.* New York: Putnam.

Thorenson, C. E. & Mahoney, M. J. (1974). *Behavioral Self-Control.* New York: Holt, Rinehart & Winston.

van Dixhoorn, J., Duivenvorden, H. J., Staal, J. A., Pool, J., & Verhage, F. (1987). Cardiac events after myocardial infarction: Possible effect of relaxation therapy. *European Heart Journal, 8.* 1210–1214.

Visintainer, M., Volpicelli, J., & Seligman, M. (1982). Tumor rejection in rats after inescapable or escapable shock. *Science, 216,* 191–199.

Watson, D. & Tharp, R. (1992). *Self-Directed Behavior: Self-Modification for Personal Adjustment,* 6th ed. Monterey, CA: Brooks/Cole. 261, 274.

Whatmore, G. B. & Kohli, D. R. (1974). *The Physiopathology and Treatment of Functional Disorders.* New York: Grune & Stratton.

Wittrock, D., Blanchard, E., & McCoy, G. (1988). Three studies on the relation of process to outcome in the treatment of essential hypertension with relaxation and thermal biofeedback. *Behaviour Research and Therapy, 26,* 53–66.

Suggested Readings on Holistic Health

Books

Achterberg, J. (1985). *Imagery in Healing: Shamanism and Modern Medicine.* Boston: New Science Library.

Achterberg, J. & Lawlis, G. F. (1978). *Imagery of Cancer.* Champaign, IL: Institute for Personality and Ability Testing.

Backhouse, K. M. & Hutchings, R. T. (1986). *Color Atlas of Surface Anatomy.* Baltimore: Williams & Wilkins.

Bailey, C. (1991). *The New Fit or Fat.* Boston: Houghton Mifflin.

Bee, H. L. (1991). *The Journey of Adulthood.* New York: Macmillan.

Benjamin, H. (1987). *From Victim to Victor.* Los Angeles: Tarcher.

Bernstein, D. A. & Borkovec, T. D. (1973). *Progressive Relaxation Training: A Manual for the Helping Professions.* Champaign, IL: Research Press.

Blake, R. (1987). *Mind over Medicine.* London: Pan Books.

Bliss, E., Bauman, E., Piper, L., Brint, A. I., & Wright, P. A. (1985). *The New Holistic Health Handbook.* New York: Viking Penguin.

Borelli, M. D. & Heidt, P. (Eds.). (1981). *Therapeutic Touch: A Book of Readings.* New York: Springer.

Borysenko, J. (1987). *Minding the Body, Mending the Mind.* Reading, MA: Addison-Wesley.

Bresler, D. (1979). *Free Yourself from Pain.* New York: Simon & Schuster.

Capacchione, L. (1988). *The Power of Your Other Hand.* North Hollywood, CA: Newcastle.

Capacchione, L. (1991). *Recovery of Your Inner Child.* New York: Simon & Schuster.

Chopra, D. (1989). *Quantum Healing.* New York: Bantam Books.

Cousins, N. (1983). *The Healing Heart.* New York: Norton.

Cousins, N. (1989). *Head First: The Biology of Hope.* New York: Dutton.

Davis, M., Eshleman, E. R., & McKay, M. (1982). *The Relaxation and Stress Reduction Workbook,* Oakland, CA: New Harbinger.

Dossey, L. (1982). *Space, Time and Medicine.* Boulder: Shambhala.

Dossey, L. (1989). *Recovering the Soul.* New York: Bantam Books.

Easwaran, E. (1981). *Dialogue with Death.* Petaluma, CA: Nilgiri Press.

Easwaran, E. (1990). *Words to Live By: Inspiration for Every Day.* Petaluma, CA: Nilgiri Press.

Ekman, P. (1985). *Telling Lies.* New York: Norton.

Feuerstein, M., Labbe, E. E., & Kuczmierczyk, A. R. (1986). *Health Psychology: A Psychobiological Perspective.* New York: Plenum.

Fiore, N. A. (1984). *The Road Back to Health.* New York: Bantam Books.

Fish, R., Weakland, J. H., & Segal, L. (1982). *The Tactics of Change.* San Francisco: Jossey-Bass.

Frank, A. W. (1991). *At the Will of the Body.* Boston: Houghton Mifflin.

Fried, R. (1990). *The Breath Connection.* New York: Plenum.

Gardner, H. (1983). *Frames of Mind.* New York: Basic Books.

Girdano, D. A., Everly, G. S., & Dusek, D. E. (1990). *Controlling Stress and Tension: A Holistic Approach* (3rd ed.). Englewood Cliffs, NJ: Prentice-Hall.

Green, E. E. & Green, A. M. (1977). *Beyond Biofeedback.* New York: Delacorte.

Hanh, T. N. (1976). *The Miracle of Mindfulness: A Manual on Meditation.* Boston: Beacon Press.

Hanh, T. N. (1987). *Being Peace.* Berkeley, CA: Parallax Press.

Hanna, T. (1988). *Somatics.* Reading, MA: Addison-Wesley.

Jacobson, E. (1974). *Progressive Relaxation* (3rd ed.). Chicago: University of Chicago Press.

Jencks, B. (1977). *Your Body Biofeedback at Its Best.* Chicago: Nelson Hall.

Jennett, B. (1986). *High Technology Medicine: Benefits and Burdens.* Cambridge: Oxford University Press.

Jones, F. P. (1976). *Body Awareness in Action.* New York: Schocken Books.

Justice, B. (1988). *Who Gets Sick: How Beliefs, Moods and Thoughts Affect Your Health.* Los Angeles: Tarcher.

Kabat-Zinn, J. (1990). *Full Catastrophe Living.* New York: Delacorte Press.

King, S. (1981). *Imagineering For Health.* Wheaton, IL: Theosophical Publishing House.

Krieger, D. (1979). *The Therapeutic Touch.* Englewood Cliffs, NJ: Prentice-Hall.

Kunz, D. (1985). *Spiritual Aspects of the Healing Arts.* Wheaton, IL: Quest Books.

Kunz, D. (1991). *The Personal Aura.* Wheaton, IL: Quest Books.

LeShan, L. (1974). *How to Meditate.* Boston: Little, Brown.

LeShan, L. (1989. *Cancer as a Turning Point.* New York: Dutton.

Levey, J. & Levey, M. (1987). *The Fine Arts of Relaxation, Concentration, and Meditation.* Boston: Wisdom.

Levine, S. (1982). *Who Dies?* New York: Anchor Books.

Levy, S. M. (1985). *Behavior and Cancer.* San Francisco: Jossey-Bass.

Lichstein, K. L. (1988). *Clinical Relaxation Strategies.* New York: Wiley.

Locke, S. & Colligan, D. (1986). *The Healer Within: The New Medicine of Mind and Body.* New York: New American Library.

Lynch, J. J. (1985). *The Language of the Heart.* New York: Basic Books.

Macrae, J. (1987). *Therapeutic Touch: A Practical Guide.* New York: Knopf.

Madanes, C. (1984). *Behind the One-Way Mirror.* San Francisco: Jossey-Bass.

Mason, L. J. (1980). *Guide to Stress Reduction.* Culver City, CA: Peace Press.

Masters, R. & Houston, J. (1978). *Listening to the Body.* New York: Delacorte Press.

Matthews-Simonton, S. (1984). *The Healing Family.* New York: Bantam Books.

McCluggage, D. (1983). *The Centered Skier.* New York: Bantam Books.

Mindell, A. (1987). *The Dreambody in Relationships.* New York: Routledge & Kegan Paul.

Nilsson, L. (1985). *The Body Victorious.* New York: Delacorte Press.

Norris, P. & Porter, G. (1985). *I Choose Life.* Walpole, NH: Stillpoint.

Nuernberger, P. (1981). *Freedom from Stress.* Honesdale, PA: Himalayan International Institute of Yoga Science and Philosophy Publishers.

Orlick, T. (1980). *In Pursuit of Excellence.* Champaign, IL: Human Kinetics.

Ornish, D. (1990). *Dr. Dean Ornish's Program for Reversing Heart Disease.* New York: Random House.

Ornstein, R. & Sobel, D. (1987). *The Healing Brain.* New York: Simon & Schuster.

Oster, G. D. & Gould, P. (1987). *Using Drawings in Assessment and Therapy.* New York: Brunner/Mazel.

Payer, L. (1988). *Medicine and Culture.* New York: Penguin Books.

Pearce, Joseph (1992). *Evaluation's End.* New York: HarperCollins.

Peck, M. S. (1978). *The Road Less Travelled.* New York: Simon & Schuster.

Pelletier, K. R. (1979). *Holistic Medicine: From Stress to Optimum Health.* New York: Delta.

Pennebaker, J. W. (1991). *Opening Up: The Healing Power of Confiding in Others.* New York: Morrow.

Peper, E. (1990). *Breathing for Health with Biofeedback.* Montreal: Thought Technology.

Peper, E., Ancoli, S., & Quinn, M. (Eds.). (1979). *Mind/Body Integration.* New York: Plenum.

Peper, E. & Williams, E. A. (1981). *From the Inside Out.* New York: Plenum.

Rama, S., Ballentine, R., & Hymes, A. (1979). *Science of Breath.* Honesdale, PA: Himalayan International Institute of Yoga Science and Philosophy Publishers.

Ritterman, M. (1983). *Using Hypnosis in Family Therapy.* San Francisco: Jossey-Bass.

Robbins, J. (1987). *Diet for a New America.* Walpole, NH: Stillpoint.

Robin, E. D. (1984). *Matters of Life and Death: Risks Versus Benefits of Medical Care.* New York: Freeman.

Rosen, S. (1982). *My Voice Will Go with You.* New York: Norton.

Rossi, E. L. (1986). *The Psychobiology of Mind–Body Healing.* New York: Norton.

Rossman, M. L. (1987). *Healing Yourself.* New York: Walker.

Sagan, L. A. (1987). *The Health of Nations: True Causes of Sickness and Well-Being.* New York: Basic Books.

Samuels, M. & Samuels, N. (1975). *Seeing with the Mind's Eye.* New York: Random House.

Schaef, A. W. (1985). *Women's Reality.* Minneapolis: Winston Press.

Seligman, M. E. P. (1991). *Learned Optimism.* New York: Knopf.

Siegel, B. S. (1986). *Love, Medicine and Miracles.* New York: Harper & Row.

Simonton, O. C., Matthews-Simonton, S., & Creighton, J. L. (1978). *Getting Well Again.* New York: Bantam Books.

Smith, M. (1975). *When I Say No, I Feel Guilty.* New York: Bantam Books.

Sobel, D. (1979). *Ways of Health.* New York: Harcourt Brace Jovanovich.

Spiro, H. M. (1986). *Doctors, Patients and Placebos.* New Haven, CT: Yale University Press.

Stroebel, C. F. (1982). *QR: The Quieting Reflex.* New York: Putnam.

Tannen, D. (1990). *You Just Don't Understand.* New York: Morrow.

Tulku, T. (1978). *Kum Nye Relaxation.* Berkeley, CA: Darma.

Vaillant, G. E. (1977). *Adaptation to Life.* Boston: Little, Brown.

Watson, D. L. & Tharp, R. G. (1981). *Self-Directed Behavior: Self-Modification for Personal Adjustment.* Monterey, CA: Brooks/Cole.

Watzlawick, P. (Ed.). (1984). *The Invented Reality.* New York: Norton.

Watzlawick, P., Weakland, J., & Fisch, R. (1974). *Change.* New York: Norton.

Wegscheider, S. (1981). *Another Chance: Hope and Health for the Alcoholic Family.* Palo Alto, CA: Science and Behavior Books.

Weil, A. (1983). *Health and Healing.* Boston: Houghton Mifflin.

Weil, A. (1990). *Natural Health: Natural Medicine.* Boston: Houghton Mifflin.

Wickramasekera, I. E. (1988). *Clinical Behavioral Medicine.* New York: Plenum.

Journals

Advances, 16E 53rd St., New York, NY 10022.

American Health, P.O. Box 3016, Harlan, IA 51593-2107.

New Sense, P.O. Box 42211, Los Angeles, CA 9042.

New Scientist, Freepost 1061, Haywards Heath, RH16 3ZA, UK

Somatics, 1516 Grant Ave., Novato, CA 94947.

Index

abuse, 141
abusive relationship, 149
accidents, automobile, 12
acne (*see* skin problems)
adaptation
    energy, 13, 15
    of self-healing strategy, 164, 174, 190–91,
        197
addictions, 142, 165, 177, 178
Ader, R., 60
adrenalin, 14
alarm reaction, 49, 50 (*see also* fight or
        flight response)
alcohol, 6, 29, 84, 142, 177, 178
Alcoholics Anonymous, 119
allergies, 14, 60, 149
amyotrophic lateral sclerosis (ALS), 150
anesthesia, 12
anger 7, 36, 79, 115, 131, 177, 183, 213
angina, 50
antidepressants, 12
antigen, 149
antihypertensive medication, 12
anxiety, 15, 117, 142, 178
    breathing and, 50
    stress and, 14

anxiety (*cont.*)
    symptoms, 50
    treatments for 50, 79, 117, 141, 177–78,
        183
art, 95, 150 (*see also* drawing; painting; mu-
        sic)
arthritis, 14
assertiveness, 7, 80, 120
asthma, 12, 14, 50, 121
    imagery and, 185
athletes, 14, 17, 95, 121, 129, 130, 163, 187
attention, 36
attitudes, 7, 115
    facilitating hand warming, 82–83
    facilitating relaxation, 26
    health and, 116, 120, 122, 184
    positive, 7, 18
attribution (*see* explanatory style)
audiotape (*see* tapes)
autogenic training, 79
automatic thoughts, 117, 122
autonomic nervous system (*see* nervous
        system)
autonomy, 9
awareness, 8, 14, 15, 17, 19, 29, 51, 71, 81–
        82, 96, 122, 162, 175, 185

225